STOP!! Killing Yourself...

The Beginners Guide to Living Longer
by Removing & Improving

RALPH MONTAGUE

This book is intended as a reference volume only, not as a medical manual.
The information given here is designed to help you make informed decisions
about your health. It is not intended as any substitute for any treatment that may
have been prescribed by your doctor. If you suspect that you have a medical
problem, we urge you to seek medical help

STOP!! Killing Yourself... first published 2020.
This edition published 2022.
© 2022 Ralph Montague
ISBN 978-1-914529-56-6
ISBN 978-1-914529-57-3

FCM Publishing

Praise for the Stop!! Workbook series

This book is dedicated to the charming and astute Peter Hill, a very fond family friend, who died during lockdown from potentially Covid-19-related symptoms, while in a specialist nursing home for dementia.

I wish that I had this knowledge and wisdom a decade ago, when I could have helped slow down Peter's rate of decline and in turn, he may not have been in the care home during lockdown.

I hope that you use the advice and knowledge in this book to help someone dear and close to you, and not just to make yourself live longer.

Table of Contents

Who This Book is For… 1

Getting Started… Living Longer Starts Here! 3

    Chapter 1 – Why I Wrote This Book 5

    Chapter 2 – Introduction to The Basics… 9

    Chapter 3 – Overview of What You Need to Do...................11

Remove… Bye, Bye Piss Stains! 13

    Chapter 4 – Remove - Sugar..15

    Chapter 5 – Remove - Stress..23

    Chapter 6 – Remove - Toxins...35

    Chapter 7 – Remove - Heat..75

    Chapter 8 – Remove - Calories 83

Improve… What's New Pussy Cat! 93

    Chapter 9 – Improve - Sleep..95

    Chapter 10 – Improve - Nutrients.....................................109

    Chapter 11 – Improve - Exercise......................................111

    Chapter 12 – Improve - Infrastructure 117

    Chapter 13 – Improve - Mind...131

Your Personalised Longevity Plan…...................................139

    Chapter 14 – Summary 141

    Chapter 15 – Give Me Five (years)… The Bare Bones Way to Live Longer! ..143

    Chapter 16 – Give Me Ten (years)… The Start of Something Great! 149

    Chapter 17 – Would You Like Any Further Help? 159

    Chapter 18 – How Ralph Can Help You?...........................161

    Chapter 19 – About the Author Ralph Montague...............163

    Chapter 20 – Further Reading & References.......................165

Index 167

WHO THIS BOOK IS FOR...

This book has been written with one end in mind, to make living longer simple to understand, with easy to follow steps.

Originally it didn't start off like this, as the sole intended reader was me. However I have now developed the thoughts and ideas a lot further, so that I have deliberately created a book that is aimed at helping:

1. **Men aged 35 to 80.**

    Although all of this information will also really help women, my experience comes purely from being a man. I can relate to what men go through and therefore have the most empathy and understanding towards them, this means that the majority of actual research undertaken has been undertaken through the male physiology.

    I believe this age range is where I can help the most, it's both early enough to create incredible lifelong habits, while still late enough to have a massive impact in the final few decades, for those who don't want to spend their last years stuck in a wheelchair, bed ridden and in agony all day long.

2. **Directors and Partners of companies.**

    Living longer has many, many side benefits. Being a director of a business for the last fifteen years, I have found the increased benefits to one's personal and business life by following these practices includes: having more energy, having a better focus, being more relaxed, finding an inner happiness, less drinking as a coping mechanism and being able to make more informed bold decisions.

Who This Book Isn't For...

- Uptight and overly sensitive people.
- Know-it-all's.
- Rude and bad-mannered people.
- Closed minded individuals.

Why? Quite frankly I would rather you carry on doing what you do and not have to deal with you as I live a longer and happier life. Of course, if you're open to change read on... if not please pass this book to someone nicer!

GETTING STARTED...
LIVING LONGER STARTS HERE!

WHY I WROTE THIS BOOK

The key to my heart has always been youthfulness and although I setup my first anti-aging and aesthetic clinic in 2005, it never even occurred to me that I could possibly ever get old. This is engrained into my very being, so much so that my reflexologist, the amazing Susana, always picks up from my feet a "Peter Pan-like" energy; her words not mine.

Over the years a lot of people have joked and said, *don't you ever age?* or *no way, you are not that old.* However, with me now being forty (no, I can't believe it either, where has all the time gone?), I thought it about time I share all the amazing things I have been doing to my body for the last twenty years, to slow down the signs of aging.

To be fair, I started off with no intention of this ever being a book, just simply, a collection of private material and research from the last twenty years. I did this in order to ensure that I continued to keep looking and feeling as great AND most importantly, as close to how I am now, both in body and mind, over the next six decades.

By understanding a little more about what I do, I hope you'll get a picture of why I wrote this book (and the forth coming sequels), or as I prefer to call them, "workbooks" as they are deliberately laid out in a format that makes you take ACTION. There is plenty of space for you to add your notes but more importantly, you need to actively use the checklists and action plans throughout the book.

I founded **The Skin Repair Clinic**, a regional chain of anti-aging aesthetic clinics back in 2005. However, I soon realised that my passion lay in researching and discovering new remarkable technologies, that help you to either feel amazing, live longer or both, and so **The Skin Repair Group** was born. It is a provider of anti-aging and longevity devices, such as cryotherapy and hyperbaric oxygen therapy.

I am also the founding partner of **The Longevity Clinic**, a central resource hub for all aspects longevity, a provider of longevity coaching, both face-to-face and a range of online courses, longevity workshops for both companies and individuals, plus advising high net-worth individuals on home longevity spas. All with the ultimate aim to help you live *"stronger for longer"*.

I even take it one significant step further and really do practice what I preach, having all this at home:

- Cryotherapy Chamber.
- Localised Cryotherapy Device.
- Hyperbaric Oxygen Chamber.
- Oxygen Facial Device.
- The Skin Repair Pen (micro needling).
- Adaptive Oxygen Therapy.
- Fat Freezing Machine.
- Red Light Therapy.
- HIFU Machine.
- HIFEM Accelerated Muscle Stimulation device.

As you can imagine, guests are both rather amused and quite stunned when they see this array of equipment, with one of the funniest moments being at 3am, managing to fit six of us in my (single use) hyperbaric oxygen chamber!!

My passion for longevity evolved when I realised '*shit, in just a few years'* *time, I was going to be forty*', having been heavily involved in the anti-ageing industry for almost two decades, it made me realise I couldn't stop time, but I could *stop* aging, well at least slow it down...

This is when the idea of **The Longevity Clinic** hit me, if I wanted to keep feeling amazing and looking a lot younger than I am, then I was sure other people would want to as well... After all, you only have to look at some of the top celebs to see what they're doing to themselves artificially in order to remain young looking.

Now I am not claiming to be a saint. I partied a lot in my twenties and early thirties and I still drink some weekends now. Ironically, it was all the partying, that was the key driver for doing everything I do and researching all these wonderful things for the human body; as I thought '*this drinking can't be good for me, just look how bad I look AND feel the next day, though I really do enjoy it, so what can I do to counter act this?*

This is when I became obsessed with all the amazing things out there that are not mainstream yet are *so*... good for us humans!

By regularly actioning the plans in this book and having the treatments at home supplied by **The Skin Repair Group**, I am walking, talking, living proof, that this stuff works incredibly and is completely safe, having been 100% tried and tested by me, on me!

Though not my first book, having also written the UK's leading aesthetics business book, **The Profitable Clinic**. this is probably the one I have enjoyed writing most. With further books in the STOP!! series to follow on sleep, energy and more advanced longevity techniques.

I hope you enjoy reading this book as much as I did writing it, however, even more importantly for me is that you action at least some of the great advice to help you live longer and stop stinking of piss at ninety.

INTRODUCTION TO THE BASICS...

I n line with the book's key objective of keeping things simple, I have written in lay terms so you can action and not get overwhelmed with words longer than the Severn Bridge!

Below are the **6 key things** you need to be paying *SUPER* attention to, in order to "Stop Killing Yourself", to live longer and not stink of piss at 90:

1. **Sleep (number 1 for a reason).**
2. **Sugar.**
3. **Stress.**
4. **Toxins.**
5. **Fasting.**
6. **Exercise.**

There are so many amazing new devices, protocols and techniques, that though the above is nowhere near an exhaustive list, if you just stick to *"Removing and Improving"* these, you will be in the top 1% of the world population, if not the top 0.1%...

It is the things that are simplest and easiest to implement that you can action today, with the biggest return on investment from both your time and money, that this book is focused on.

What this book is NOT about, is giving you the most complicated and expensive cutting-edge treatments, that will make you live to 1,000 years old!

That's not to say there won't be a part two, as there is and in fact a part four planned in the STOP!! series, but that's only for those who want to live to 500 years' old. So, let's stick to the basics first and get you started on this living stronger for longer trip, or "youngevity" as I also like to call it.

OVERVIEW OF WHAT YOU NEED TO DO 3

This book has been written in a simple set format, whereby each chapter will visit a key topic, in your quest for being super active and healthy at ninety and if you're lucky (which I know you are) even getting the occasional leg over, once in a while!

I aim to explain why each aspect/character is important with a background of the issue without boring the hell out of you and trying to impress you with overly long words and technical jargon. I am guessing for most of you, this doesn't matter and you simply want to feel marvellous and live longer, I get it!

Next, this is the part where "you" are going to do some work! For every chapter you and I are to visit together, I have created your personalised fact finder to follow, this NEEDS TO BE DONE. No tomorrow, no later, no ifs, no buts and if you don't want to do it, I'd rather you don't bother reading this book anymore and give it to someone who will do these fact finds!

Please action these points, as I want you to feel better. Though why do I care? Well, when you feel better, you will tell other people how amazing you feel, and in turn more people will buy this book, which helps me to step back from work and write more books. I did ask my parents if I could retire and live with them rent free, so I could spend my days writing and researching, but they said no, so I still have to work to pay the bills, (rude!) so please tell people about this book, if you've benefited from it!

For each point, I have written a brief summary of why this is important and what you can do to either "Remove or Improve".

Then finally, the third part brings everything together, in a simple and easy to follow action plan, that you can work through to create a longer living and younger you.

The book really is that simple… you can thank me when you are ninety going on sixty. Please note, I am also open to gifts from grateful and healthy ninety year old's who have read my book; small tokens such as week long trips on your super yacht, Rolls Royce convertibles, Patek Phillipe watches etc…

It's on this note that I remind you of the network effect of longevity and living longer. It's no good doing this alone, and getting to watch your wife/husband, children, siblings and many great friends all die many years before you, leaving you alone at a stage in life where it might not be as easy to make new connections and certainly not ones as meaningful (unless of course they're in my list of people who shouldn't read this book and in which case, maybe have a life laundry too!).

It's for this reason, that I urge you to share what you learn in this book with those close to you, get them involved and make it a fun activity, so that you all benefit together.

On a completely selfish note for you to finally consider, it will also save you having to wipe their arse when they are old and decrepit! Nothing like self-interest now is there…

REMOVE...
BYE, BYE PISS STAINS!

REMOVE - SUGAR 4

From a young age we are all told not to smoke, drink and take drugs yet for a long time no one really warned us against one of the world's biggest "silent killers" SUGAR!

This stuff really is horrific for us humans. *Why is it that bad*? I can hear you all say. Well, it's all to do with inflammation, which is the root cause to the world's most "popular", hard to treat, yet easiest to prevent, chronic diseases, such as;

- Heart disease.
- Cancer.
- Diabetes.
- Alzheimer's.
- Lung disease.
- Strokes.

And what is one of the most "popular" root causes of inflammation…you guessed it, processed sugar. We will also cover in the next chapter, the other key factor in inflammation, stress. So, by simply removing sugar and stress from your life, you have created life changing habits, that will see you living a lot longer and a lot healthier life, or as I like to call it "stronger for longer".

Inflammation is not intended to be bad for you, in fact quite the opposite, as it's the bodies healing mechanism to fix you if something goes wrong. For example, if you get cut, the body via the immune system releases an array of response reactions to instigate the healing process. You will often notice this taking place by the said area being warm, red and swollen, this is inflammation.

However, the problem with inflammation is not the occasional response to an issue, it's the on-going continuous exposure of our bodies to inflammation - that's the big concern. It's this permanent or chronic inflammation, that is at the heart of every long-term illness.

If we take the world's most "popular" chronic disease, heart disease, this is caused mainly by inflammation of the arteries, which also helps you on your way to get diabetes and a stroke…

Obviously, there are other contributors, however sugar is a great starting point in line with this book's philosophy of keeping things simple. That being said we will cover these in the later chapters.

The purpose of this chapter is to get you to stop taking sugar. Yes, I term it that way, like you would say to an addict, "stop taking heroin".

Before we go through all the ways to help you get off sugar, let's do a little fact find, to see just how sweet, you really are…

How Sweet Are You?

1. Do you add sugar or any other sweetener to your drinks e.g. tea or coffee?

    ....

    ....

    ....

2. Do you drink fizzy soft drinks e.g. coke and if so, how often?

    ....

    ....

    ....

3. Do you have deserts after dinner and if so, how often?

    ....

    ....

    ....

4. In the day, will you have biscuits, doughnuts, cakes etc. mid-morning or afternoon?

    ....

    ....

    ....

5. Do you ever check the sugar level on packaged foods?

....

....

....

Stop Being So Sweet...

One of the first things you have to do, if you are serious about living longer, is start to lower your sugar intake. Don't do this all at once, otherwise you might be less inclined to stick with your great new habit.

If you take two sugars (teaspoons) with your tea, just drop this down to one sugar for the next few weeks and it won't be long before you get used to this and one sugar, becomes your new norm.

Then once you are used to one sugar, drop that down to half a sugar, then after a few weeks you can either remove the sugar completely or take it down to a quarter, if you are still clutching on to your old ways.

Any reduction in your current consumption is great, so though the goal is to not adding ANY sugar, even if you just halve your sugar intake, I'm a happy man. Also very happy, is your body, with this being a very strong move forward for you.

No level of soft drink is good for you, a typical can of Coke contains 36 grams of sugar and guess what the American Heart Association's recommended daily sugar level is for an adult? You guessed it, the very same, well 1 gram more at 37 grams per day.

So, by having just one can of Coke, you are maxing out on your entire sugar intake, for that day. When put like that, do you still want that Coke?

The only solution here, is to stop drinking soft drinks or as I like to call them, carbonated sugar!

Just in case you think I'm biased, Dr Pepper has 24g and Sprite 34g.

I always remember a guy I used to work with in one of my first jobs after uni, he drank around 1.5 litres of Coke, religiously every day, not only that, but he would also brag about it at work events over a few beers. He looked terrible, he was in his mid 30s yet already looked down and out with brown teeth, dull rotting skin and he wondered why he was single…

However, in line with getting optimum uptake from you, if you are currently drinking a can a day, reduce this to a can every other day, for a few weeks and then after a month or so, you will be easily able to take this down to just one a week Before long, you will simply stop craving it and can remove it completely from your life, for good. You may also find that after removing it from your diet, if you have one at a party it'll be way too sweet for you.

This next bit was probably the hardest for me, having grown up with ice cream every night after din dins! In the last decade, I have stopped buying ice cream every weekly shop and limited it to just once a month, when I would treat myself. However, in the last year, now knowing just how incredibly bad sugar is (I always knew it was bad, just didn't realise, it was this bad!) I have even stopped my monthly treat, so no ice cream for Ralphy (never said this was going to be easy!). However, it was a lot easier to give up than I realised, as now I don't get that horrible dairy after taste in my mouth all night anymore, no weird changes in my mood or being bloated.

If you are having desserts with your evening meal every night, then why don't you just make it a treat, once a week for Friday after the end of a week of work? Or perhaps Saturday night, when you go out for dinner with friends?

You don't have to quit desserts completely (though this would be great if you did), just limit the times you have them, to special occasions.

This next one, is a killer for your productivity and mood throughout the day! The mid-morning or afternoon tea break, with biscuits, cakes or dare I say it, doughnuts!

I can't even be bothered to ask you nicely to gradually reduce this habit, just stop and stop now. You do not realise, what a huge impact this is having on your life.

Biscuits have everything in life you don't want in something that goes in your mouth. First off, it's not food. Its highly processed junk food, then we have the sugar/high carbs, the vegetable oils, the white flour, and if all that wasn't enough all the preservatives.

Finally, it's worth checking the labels of food you think is safe to eat, I was absolutely overwhelmed when I checked the sugar content in ketchup, luckily, we don't have that much in a serving.

The other items that I know aren't ideal, though thought were ok, like a McDonald's iced frappe - yes, I do still occasionally go to Maccy D's as it can be convenient when on the road and hungry, even though I know it's terrible, hence why its limited to such "emergencies"!

This is the theme and point behind this book, you don't have to remove things completely or forever, it's more about limiting the frequency and/or the amount you have. I was actually horrified when found out that there is 88g of sugar in a MacDonald's iced frappe, that's almost three days of sugar in one drink!

REMOVE - STRESS 5

Another silent assassin, that's all around us…

Just look at the defensive way people these days react to any confrontation, or the quick to react road rage, never mind the whole world being so uptight and sensitive to any (perceived) insult. Well, this is the cumulation of years of stress with no form of release, pent up inside, ready to explode and explode it does! Just look at social media, for all the continuous stream of 'outraged' people…

Humans today are trying to cope with the increased stress levels, the modern (western) world has brought us. We are not designed for this new modern world, full of 24/7 bright lights, continuous alerts, combined with all the hustle and bustle.

Just think of what most of us have to go through day-to-day in life:

- Bringing up children.
- Work deadlines.
- Mortgage/rent payments.
- Health worries.
- Looking after elderly parents (a lot with dementia and other serious health concerns).
- Being contactable 24 hours a day.

- Continuous beeping of alerts going off.
- Commuting.
- Fear of crime/violence.
- Plus, I am sure you have your own personal stresses…

My first real encounter of stress was my dad's attitude towards me on a regular basis, when I moved back home after uni and was travelling for my first job.

After a long day in work, I would come home to my sister and I, constantly being berated for various things. Looking back now, it is actually quite amusing, however, at the time, it was a constant bombardment of stress on all fronts, without a calm environment to relax in.

Before long, this brought me out in psoriasis. At first, I was massively confused as to why I had these unsightly red patches of skin on my hands. I even went to the doctors about it and was given a range of things that didn't work, before finally being given steroid cream that improved the symptoms, though not eliminating them and most importantly, still did not fix the cause.

One thing I have learnt in life is prevention is better than cure, from watching the health issues of my mother, who spends a lot of her time "trying" to fix problems that sadly now can't be fixed and at best are just mildly improved. Nevermind the pain, energy and loss of experiencing life. Bad decisions just like good decisions compound.

A year later, the most interesting thing happened however, I sold my beautiful Alfa Romeo GTV (so painful!), to buy my first house. Then, in a matter of just a few days, the patchy red scaly skin, just disappeared. It was then, that I realised the power that stress has on, not just our mental wellbeing, but also, also our physical wellbeing.

Stress really is a killer, a silent killer!

Every time you get stressed, you are taking a small amount of time from your life. It continuously wears you down, slowly but very surely. Along with sugar, stress is the key contributor to inflammation and as we have covered, the root causes to the world's most popular killers.

So how does stress kill us silently? It's mainly (though not all) to do with two hormones, cortisol and adrenaline.

Cortisol is produced by the adrenal glands and is a very, very important hormone for us humans. Though it's often thought of as bad, we need cortisol to perform properly, it's just that too much cortisol, is bad for us and so is, too little!

If we have too little cortisol, when we wake up in the morning, we will feel tired, even after a long sleep, as we need the cortisol to wake us up. Stress can burn out our cortisol reserves, which in turn makes us tired when we first wake.

Even worse is that if you have too little cortisol, you lose its anti-inflammatory benefits, that create excess inflammation, which can lead to a number of health issues, such as rheumatoid arthritis.

It's the turning of proteins in the muscle to glucose that causes the serious and long-term health issues. This is what too much cortisol does, by increasing your blood glucose level, if you are constantly stressed. This then leads to increased weight gain, heightened risk of diabetes and/or heart attacks.

Adrenaline on the other hand, tells the body when to release glucose into the blood stream, in order to fuel your body with the energy needed if you have to fight or flight, speeding up your heart rate, which I'm sure you have all experienced at some point in your life.

It's this continuous state of being on guard that the modern western world, i.e. toxic, anti-social media, twenty-four-hour fear based news and attention consuming tech, has created for us, which is why what is actually designed to be a good and safe bodily reaction/function, is actually harming us.

Very interesting however, is that the end game of stress comes back to sugar/glucose levels in the blood…

How Stressed Are You?

1. How many nights a week do you wake up in the middle of the night, with a lot on your mind?

    ....

    ....

    ....

2. Do you find yourself getting angry quickly and/or over minor things?

    ....

    ....

    ....

3. Do you worry about the future or are you a worrier in general?

    ....

    ....

    ....

4. Do YOU dictate what happens to you, or do you let the WORLD dictate what happens to you?

    ....

    ....

    ....

5. Are you worrying continuously about your children?

    ....

    ....

    ....

6. Are you spending a lot of time on your phone replying to texts, social media notification and emails, yet still can't manage to get through them all?

    ....

    ....

    ....

7. Do you feel overwhelmed with life?

    ....

    ....

    ....

8. Do you have financial worries?

    ....

    ....

    ....

9. Do you find going to work a chore and something you don't actually look forward to?

    ....

    ....

    ....

10. Do you have any health concerns and if so what?

    ....

    ....

    ....

11. Does the state of the world or your country really get to you?

    ....

    ....

    ....

12. Do you rely on coffee and/or Red Bull type energy drinks throughout the day to get you going, yet then at night in order sleep resort to a few alcoholic drinks?

    ....

    ....

    ....

13. If you commute, how do you feel about it?

....

....

....

Your Personal Notes

Time to Calm it Down...

The solution to all of these is really quite simple!

The first course of action for you would be to exercise, as this burns off anxiety and worry. It really is a game changer, regardless of all the other amazing health benefits you get from exercise.

Next would be to stop all stimulants after 2pm, ideally midday, however 2pm will allow you to see drastic improvements in your ability to sleep and relax come the evening (and not require booze).

Stop worrying about things in your life you can't control e.g. the state of the economy or terrorism, and just focus on what you CAN control. This has a powerful effect on your mind. First, you are no longer wasting valuable time and energy on things you have little or no influence on, so they are best simply forgotten about. Next by focusing on what you can control, it gives you a great sense of direction and a say in your life.

Do not underestimate the big impact that simply being amongst nature can have on reducing your stress. Being by the sea, which is my favourite, provides you with lots of negative ions, that are simply amazing for you, plus there's the calming sound of the waves, which subconsciously help you to regulate your breathing. There is the forest or mountains, whereby you get the phytoncide from trees and in fact in Japan, they even refer to it as 'forest bathing', due to all the goodness you get from nature.

Finally, put those bloody phones away! Turn off your notifications on your phone, for everything, except perhaps phone calls (the original purpose of a phone). This means beeps, vibrations and flashing lights, so no distraction. By constantly being interrupted by this modern cancer, you are putting yourself under lots of minor stress continuously throughout the day.

For the super brave out there (perhaps only SAS and Seals are brave enough for this one!), turn off your phone an hour before you go to bed, then turn it back on again at midday, the following day. I do this around 4 or 5 times a week and it's amazing how much you get done.

In fact, it's really weird, as you end up getting lots of work done to a high standard, yet it feels almost effortless and that you haven't actually worked that hard at all.

The other added benefit of this, is that you don't get the crazy idiots who keep calling you multiple times when you don't answer the first time, as you are busy (odd I know during a working day).

They now won't be able to ring you twenty times, in the space of just a few hours! I've now started blocking these annoying and selfish individuals. Whatever happened to the old, call once, maybe even twice, later in the day, leave a voice message and the person calls you back after their meeting?

I now simply remove anyone like this from my life, these people are killing you by the stress and drama they create and cause. Remove them from your life, or they remove your life from you.

Plus, rather ironically, they often block you when you are no longer any use to them and they don't need you anymore!

A super easy and quick win is to just simply turn off the news, for those worried about the world and their country, this is one of the worst things you can be consuming. Just turn it off!

Plus, you will also be very grateful for the time you save. As those into the news, will watch it typically daily and if you think thirty mins a day, which is easily done, works out at nine hundred minutes a month, which adds up to fifteen hours, or two average working days given back to you, every single month. However, when you look at it from an entire life perspective, the figures just blow your mind as it equates to two-thousand-four-hundred working days over a hundred year life (yes, I know babies don't watch the news, however it kept the maths simple!).

Just think of how less stressful your life would be with all this extra time to get things done, plus you've also now recouped all that wasted time, worrying about things you can't even control, as that worry has now simply disappeared!

This is a beginner's guide to living longer, so I don't want to go into meditation too much, (plus it's in the next books and I don't want to spoil that). However, if you already do this, then incorporate it into a daily habit, to help you reduce your stress levels.

Sleep is key to you being a lot calmer and less stressed. Plus, the good news is, we have a whole chapter on this, coming up shortly for you…

So, in order to live a stress-free life, well a life with a lot less stress, as for us humans, there is no avoiding stress completely, the above are very simple and yet quick wins for you.

REMOVE - TOXINS 6

This chapter was the reason for the title of this book, STOP!! Killing Yourself..., I originally wanted to call the book "*Stop Stinking of Piss at 90 & Start Shagging Again!*", however, one of my best friends quickly pointed out, that very few people would be happy to read such a book on a train, bus, plane or generally in public!

Also, this is my favourite topic and therefore not surprisingly, the first chapter I wrote (yes that's right, I started writing chapter 6 before chapter 1). It's so fascinating when you start to scratch the surface, of the *huge* lies we have continuously been told and the horrifically dangerous substances we come into contact with on a daily basis, yet are never actually told just how bad these things are for us.

Has it ever crossed your mind just how toxic and dangerous your daily walk to work along that busy road in your polluted city is? Or what the fumes from the carpet in your bedroom may be doing to you, while you sleep every night, whilst also being surrounded by city centre pollution!

The reason toxins are so key to your longevity, is the damage and extra workload they place on your liver. A toxin is merely a substance that damages your body in some way.

Some are blatantly obvious, like cigarettes, while others are more silent and hidden, like the lead paint on your walls or the Botox, ironically injected into you to make you look "younger".

All however are putting extra stress on your liver and like the rest of you, your liver is also aging and becoming less efficient, every year we occupy a space on this planet, and it's for that reason we need to be as kind as truly possible to this organ, as the liver is key, to keeping you alive and still shagging at ninety!

As my plan is to make this more of an actionable book, than a sit back and relax book, I am going to get straight into your personal toxin's consultation…

I've divided the toxins into categories to make things easier for you, which are:

1. **People.**
2. **Home.**
3. **Daily Routine.**
4. **Environment.**
5. **Work.**
6. **Orally.**

Your Toxic Checklist...

<u>People</u>

1. Do you lose your temper or get angry, more than twice a week with the people you live with?

    ....

    ....

    ....

2. Do you lose your temper or get angry more than twice a week with the people you work with?

    ....

    ....

    ....

3. How long do you typically remain angry for, is it often for more than just a few moments, i.e. longer than 5 minutes?

    ....

    ....

    ....

4. Do you hate anyone you have to work with e.g. colleagues, customers or suppliers?

....

....

....

5. Write a list of all your friends you regularly see (at least once a quarter), then put a line through those that have caused problems twice or more in the last year. Remember, friendships should be enjoyable and supportive not toxic and draining, while appreciating we all need support and compassion from time to time!

....

....

....

6. Have you fallen out with any of your neighbours?

....

....

....

Your Personal Notes

Home

1. Do your household fabrics e.g. carpets, curtains, sofas etc. contain volatile organic matter (VOC)? You probably don't know, however it's worth you finding out.

    ....

    ....

    ....

2. Does your paint contain lead? Again, unless you did this yourself, you probably don't know, however this is worth finding out!

    ....

    ....

    ....

3. Are the water pipes into your house lead (will only apply to old houses built before 1970s)? This a bit easier to know or find out.

    ....

    ....

    ....

4. Do you use a chemical disinfectant in the kitchen and bathrooms? I know the answer to this will be yes for 99% of you!

    ....

    ....

    ....

5. Do you have air fresheners or sprays around the house?

   ....

   ....

   ....

6. What chemicals are in the capsules/tablets/powder you use to wash your clothes? Are you getting irritated skin, could it be your detergent?

   ....

   ....

   ....

7. Do you keep your mobile phone on your person at all times throughout the day?

   ....

   ....

   ....

8. Do your lights emit UV light?

   ....

   ....

   ....

9. Do you sleep with your mobile phone next to your brain?

....

....

....

10. Is your WI-FI left on overnight?

....

....

....

11. Do you sleep with synthetic and potentially chemical ridden pillows or duvets?

....

....

....

Daily Routines

1. What's in your toothpaste, fluoride (one of my best friends, an expert dentist, would argue with me on this point and he has good points, however this is my book, so bugger off Russell!)?

    ....

    ....

    ....

2. Do you use an aerosol spray deodorant?

    ....

    ....

    ....

3. Do you use a natural deodorant or one with toxic aluminium in (I am a hypocrite here, however will explain why, in the next section)?

    ....

    ....

    ....

4. Do you use an aerosol hair spray?

    ....

    ....

    ....

5. Do you know what's in your makeup and moisturisers? Well now's the time to check those ingredients…

    ....

    ....

    ....

6. Same goes for your shower gel, handwash, shampoo and conditioner, what chemicals are you putting into contact with your body every day?

    ....

    ....

    ....

Your Personal Notes

<u>Environment</u>

1. Do you live on or near a busy road?

    ....

    ....

    ....

2. Do you live next to any transport hubs e.g. airports or train stations?

    ....

    ....

    ....

3. Do you walk/run/cycle to work or exercise along a busy road?

    ....

    ....

    ....

4. Do you live near a factory pumping out pollution?

    ....

    ....

    ....

5. Do you live under or near electricity lines?

    ....

    ....

    ....

6. Do any of your neighbours generate excessive noise that irritates you on a regular basis?

    ....

    ....

    ....

Work

1. Can you open the windows in your office?

    ....

    ....

    ....

2. Does the air feel stuffy or static and just generally yuck?

    ....

    ....

    ....

3. What chemicals do you come into contact with during your job? Have you personally checked if these are harmful and please don't just take your employer's word for it!

    ....

    ....

    ....

4. Is there a nice environment/energy in your workplace or is it hostile, uptight, quiet etc?

    ....

    ....

    ....

5. A lot of the issues for your home are the same issues in your workplace, however for most people you have little control over these at work, unless you are a director or owner of the business hence why not revisited here. But if you can change these aspects, then please do so for your own health's sake and your fellow colleagues. Refer back to the home section to revisit these aspects.

    ....

    ....

    ....

Your Personal Notes

Orally

1. Do you smoke?

    ....

    ....

    ....

2. Do you drink daily?

    ....

    ....

    ....

3. How often do you get actually tipsy/drunk?

    ....

    ....

    ....

4. Though sugar has its very own chapter, as it's that horrifically bad for you, I am briefly mentioning it here, as another reminder to get sugar out of your fucking life!! How many grams of sugar a day do you have?

    ....

    ....

    ....

5. Do you buy organic food, if so, how much is organic as a percentage of your food shop?

....

....

....

6. How many meals a week do you eat that need the top pricking with a fork?

....

....

....

7. Do you store your liquids and food in plastics? This includes pre-packaged water?

....

....

....

8. Do you filter your tap water?

....

....

....

Your Personal Notes

Time to Review Your Answers & Your Action Plan...

To keep things simple, I have kept the explanations below brief for each section, in order to not overwhelm you with another 40 or so points! However, at the end of the book I have put together longevity action plans for you based on the below, with options depending on the level of effort you are wanting to put into living longer.

People

Like sugar, stress has its very own chapter however due to how they are both in the "Top 5 Super Removers" I have deliberately brought this up again, as there is nothing like repetition, to hammer home an important point!

If you are finding yourself angry multiple times a week and/or for long periods of time, this is going to make you ill. And when I mean ill, not some cold (though it does reduce your immune system and you will get more annoying colds), we are talking serious chronic illness, like strokes, heart attacks, cancer and diabetes, to name but a few!

You have a few options to overcome this, firstly it's most likely you, if this is happening a lot and with numerous different people.

You can either deny it as you are perfect and be in both long term chronic pain AND then (it gets even better!) be the most righteous man in the graveyard OR, think fuck having to be right all the time, I'd rather feel happy, healthy and see my (great) grandchildren get married and have their first child!

However, there are times when you are simply surrounded by some of the most awkward, stubborn bastards this world has ever produced, and I appreciate there are a lot of them out there!

As much as I love my father very dearly, he sometimes can be such a man, things like going out for a meal, to putting new towels out when I stay, have caused huge arguments and he is always right, of course! So be aware, some of the people you love most in the world, can be contributing to your early death…

In these cases, like I do with my dad, I simply only see him once a fortnite now as he is my dad and I love him very much I can't not see him. However, often I will come away from seeing him and my mood has changed for the worst, I feel tension inside me and can even feel fucked off. This is not good for my health so I "Remove" this toxicity from my life as best as I can, yet it's not easy, I can grant you that!

Now if these are a colleague, member of staff or a lover, then it gets even simpler as you can quit, sack, or dump them! It may take a bit of time to manoeuvre your situation, however it can be done and *needs* to be done… soon.

Neighbours is an interesting one… as you can be all chummy one day, then all of a sudden, for example you don't mow your lawn when they want you to, (I have first-hand experience of this one!) then those twice a week, half an hour, pleasant conversations you always have, turn into that same person completely blanking you. Now it took me weeks to work out the sudden split personality of the said neighbour opposite, and though still not sure, this seems to be the most likely case…

Now I could confront him, this could easily escalate into an argument and then all sorts of funny games to get one up on each other… OR you can simply ignore him and carry on with a calm peaceful life!

However, so many people refuse to let things go! This is doing you so much harm to your own health, in fact they are helping to kill you, so each time you want to react, just remember do you want them to slowly kill you!

It's worth noting he doesn't speak with his next-door neighbour either, so always a good move to spot these people early on as they can become your silent assassin, if you enter into their funny world of grudges and games…

Finally, friends! Or as some can be more like silent enemies. You will find that out of your group of friends, some people just cause problems, they attract them all the bloody time!

I used to have a friend Larry (not his real name) and he was always asking to borrow money, late for work, getting sacked, problems with where he was living etc, the list was endless…

I really liked Larry and thoroughly enjoyed spending time with him, as we would have such a great laugh together, however, it wasn't until my new girlfriend said to me, *"has it not dawned on you all the problems Larry brings you"*? and though I was aware, it had never crossed my mind that I didn't have to be friends with him and I could simply remove him from my life, so I did.

It was relatively easy as he owed me £80, so I asked for this back, he said he didn't have it and I knew that this was going to turn into one of my greatest investments ever, by simply letting him keep the £80. In return, I wouldn't hear from him and I didn't for about two years, until he called, so I asked him for the money back he owed me, he claimed he was skint (he always is) and I've not heard from him since and that was 8 years ago!

Perfect, if I can do it, then so can you.

<u>Home</u>

We now look back at the Victorians and laugh at the fact that they used to have arsenic in their paint! However, there is a huge lesson here… does it not make you think if the Victorians were happy to put arsenic on their walls back then, what are we consuming today, that people in a hundred years will look back on and laugh at us?

Don't be fooled to think it can't happen to us, as it will happen, and we will be very surprised at some of these instances! On the other hand, they will be in stitches at the fact we used to have such highly insulated houses, with no ventilation and then wonder why we had such bad health...

I am super anal when it comes to painting of doors, skirting boards and wood in general. I actually leave the house, as the toxic smell is just too much and if at all possible, will even stay away for a few days afterwards (though annoyingly this is not always possible) due to the toxic lingering fumes.

Before painting, look for good quality safe paints and be very careful what you are putting on your walls!

The same goes for fabrics in your house, the chemicals used to treat your carpet, sofa and curtains can be quite toxic in some cases and you really need to understand what you are buying, and how it's been treated.

Water is one of my favourites. I just love water, this means I like my water to be in a safe state when it arrives at my lips. If I am ever eating out in an old building, as most are in the beautiful Regency town of Cheltenham, this mean that there is a very good chance that the plumbing is still very old and pre 1970's.

Though not always the case, as if refurbing a restaurant, it would make perfect sense to upgrade the plumbing at the same time, however that being said there is no real way for me to find this out, without pulling tiles off the wall when I go for a pee! So, I always edge on the side of caution and won't *ever* drink their tap water, instead I opt for spring/mineral water in a glass bottle.

When it comes to your house, it's worth checking the plumbing. If you live in an old house and if you have lead pipes (low chance though possible) get these changed *yesterday*, as the water will be killing you when you shower, even if you filter all your drinking water, (as you should be wherever you live).

That being said there is one aspect that you can't do much about, and that's external plumbing. I dealt with this in a previous house, one that was built in the 1890's. As we were going through the renovations, I could see the pipes connecting my house to the water mains were lead. Oh shit! However, bugger all I could do about it, my only options were move or harass the local water board to get it changed, who let's be honest, wouldn't be particularly interested in replacing this...

Disinfectant sprays are an interesting one, we generally apply these with a spray mechanism, allowing these toxic chemicals, which bad enough are going on your hands when wiping down surfaces, yet on top of this, you are sending these toxic chemicals into the air and then inhaling them, when you breath! So, if it's not being absorbed through your skin or via any cuts on your hands, it's also coming in via your lungs.

Hydrogen peroxide seems to be the best natural alternative so far, though I explore this further in an article on my website:

www.thelongevityclinic.co.uk.

Alternatively, you could consider a toxin free alternative:

A great all-purpose cleaner from disinfectant sprays to floor wash to toilet cleaner, is to mix two cups of water with one cup of cider vinegar, this is a thorough, sturdy cleaner that can get rid of everything from grease and stains to mildew and mould. Add a few drops of an essential oil of your choice to give it a clean scent, ie: lemongrass, or eucalyptus.

The same goes as above, when it comes to air fresheners. How about just opening the window? So, what if it's cold outside, the cold is good for you, never mind the benefits of the fresh air and the removal of positive ions generated from your electrical appliances.

A handy, toxin-free alternative is to mix ten drops of essential oil with half a cup of water to a spray bottle and you have a homemade, cost-effective, toxic-free air freshener. It's important to use a 100% pure essential oil for maximum scent, and no nasties in the mix.

Mobile phones are covered in the chapter on stress, however here, we look at them from the other angle whereby they directly kill us, as opposed to just indirectly. The EMF (electromagnetic fields) radiation phones give off are not kind on human's soft tissue. Ask yourself, how does your ear (and brain) feel after a 15 minute plus phone call on your mobile when held against your head? Exactly, your head is super-hot and feels like it's going to explode!

I mainly take phone calls on my mobile, using a set of "wired" headphones and NOT the blue tooth headphones. Otherwise, I am again exposing myself to more EMF radiation, albeit a lot less, though akin to replacing a broken foot with a broken toe! Why break anything! If I don't have a set of headphones with me (spare set in car, spare set in briefcase and spare set in my office) then I will take calls on loudspeaker, with the phone around 25cms away from my head.

Another thing I started a few months back and yet knew I should have done this about 5 years ago (though in my defence I have been putting my phone on aeroplane mode for almost a decade now), was to remove my phone charger from my bedroom and place this in my office (if you don't have an office, this can be downstairs in your living room - however if you are having an affair this could prove the end of your marriage I appreciate, which would be more stressful, so then please just keep your phone next to you, frazzling your brain, I just hope she's worth it!).

This has so many benefits, stress reduction, sleep improvement and no frying of the brain!

I've said for a very long time, way before any scientific proof had confirmed this, that this can't be good for our brains, being surrounded by yet another source of EMF radiation, I just had a gut feeling. Now numerous studies have shown this to be the case. I believe we all need to be protecting ourselves from this serious harm.

Though some studies have shown it to be safe, they generally have some financial incentive behind the scenes, from the industry most likely to lose out if this is widely known. Just think of big tobacco claiming cigarettes are safe and Camels claim that it was the doctors preferred cigarette! You laugh but all this actually happened…

A simple solution and one that I adopt, is to simply just turn off my Wi-Fi when I am not using it. It started off just overnight however, I am now getting into the habit of turning it off when it's not needed i.e. not using it (the other benefit is it stops pings coming through and distracting e.g. emails, WhatsApp, notification on anti-social media etc.)

For a lot of people with sensitive skin, who have been searching for years to the source of their irritable skin and red rashes, it comes as a big surprise to them, to find out it's their washing powder! The very stuff that is supposed to be keeping them clean! For this book I took one of my Persil capsules and broke the liquid out on to my hands and my God, were they super itchy and irritated (yes, I know it says not to get in contact with the skin on the packaging), plus I appreciate these capsules are significantly diluted with lots of water when put in the washing machine, however it certainly gets you thinking…

A girlfriend of mine was very sensitive to a lot of things in life (probably me as well!) and she would have to wash her clothes with a special detergent, for these very reasons. It would be worth edging on the side of caution and using non-bio washing detergents as you then don't have the enzymes in, which are used to digest the stains in clothes and cause the irritability.

It may be worth trying a plant-based laundry option, these will be toxin free and more environmentally friendly (no point in living longer if it's on a destroyed planet), there are many on the market and cut out all the hazardous ingredients used in most household laundry detergents.

On that note, I always used to find it hilarious that if you bought my mum anything not gold or silver i.e. some plated cheap crap, she would literally come out in a rash! Clever mum…

If you think about it, clothes are in continuous contact with your body and if they are laced with strong chemicals this could be causing you problems, I personally have no (visible) problems however now that I have just turned 40, it's time for me to change as like with a lot of these toxins, a lot is lurking inside that we can't see or even feel, and we only find out to our peril, when things start going wrong...

When it comes to nearly everything in life, if there is a natural alternative, I always go with the natural option and bedding is no different. For that reason, always opt for natural bedding so that's cotton, wool and feathers. My pillows and duvets are all Hungarian Down feathers and not manmade foams, very deliberately.

However, I appreciate some people have allergies to such fillings and are unable to have these. What is super interesting about that last statement, is that when you start actioning the steps in this book, you will find you no longer actually have a lot of these allergies and can now in fact sleep with the best feathers in town!

Finally, give a thought to the type of lighting you have in your home, the new style, uber powerful (and fashionable) spotlights provide us with a bright white/blue light which is great in the morning when we want to wake up, yet really bad for our sleep pattern in the evening (this is covered in the chapter on sleep which is very important, so have brought it up once more as a gentle reminder).

On top of this and the key aspect for this chapter, is that internal lighting can emit higher than ideal UV light which in excess is bad for us and has been linked to skin cancer. So again, this is worth checking out if you spend a lot of time indoors!

Routine

There is a lot of controversy over fluoride, as on one hand it helps against tooth decay, while on the other, too much fluoride can be toxic.

My toothpaste doesn't have fluoride, it's aloe vera based and it is as natural as possible, considering it comes in a plastic tube! I explore the fluoride debate further in an article I have written which you can read at www.thelongevityclinic.co.uk. A handy natural mouthwash to have at home is coconut oil. Swish a small spoonful of the stuff for approx one minute in the morning and at night for stain free, plaque resistant gnashers!

When in school, getting changed after PE (physical education) lessons, it always dawned on me that all the multiple sprays going around the changing room from everyone's deodorant, was incredibly intoxicating and thought to myself surely this can't be good for anyone's health here.

My (occasionally smelly) dad who refuses to wear deodorant, was banging on about the fumes from the aerosols decades ago. Though mum and I agreed with him, we still suggested he should use a roll-on deodorant as occasionally it could be a little embarrassing the waft of body odour!

That being said Big Will was right and from a young age, I switched to roll on deodorants for this very reason, while all my friends were silently intoxicating themselves, in their cramped bedrooms full of fumes. Where possible, I remove myself instantly from a room full of aerosol fumes!

For years I thought I was pretty fly for a white guy being one step ahead when it came to deodorants, then I watched a documentary back in 2017 on aluminium production (yes, I must have been super bored that day I know, well hungover!), WOW, my eyes were opened up, well and truly, to this toxic metal.

And guess what's in deodorant… you got it! Aluminium.

So, for the next year I tested a few different "natural" deodorants and some which were super safe, resulted in me stinking like my dad, not good…especially on dates! A few others left me with severe itching (again not good being in public frantically scratching your armpits, people might start throwing bananas at you!).

It took some time to find both a natural deodorant that stopped me stinking and was kind to my body.

However, I'm still trialling what works best for me. I'm yet to find the right one, so if there's anyone out there that wants to recommend something, I'm open to suggestions.

The same goes for hair spray, as this is an aerosol, due to this I tend to use a gum, so that no sprays are used in my bathroom at all. Around one in three UK adults have some form of allergic disease and these can be aggravated by aerosols.

Even for those without allergies, you are still exposing yourself to the risk of headaches, breathing issues and skin reactions, due to the fact that you will most likely be applying these in a small, confined space i.e. your bathroom (doors and windows will most likely be shut and a lot of ensuite or apartment bathrooms don't even have windows) and the fine mist is not just easily inhaled, it actually lingers in the air, easily facilitating its inhalation!

And finally, do you really want high levels of butane and propane in your blood long term!

I would also read the labels on the back of your makeup and moisturisers? You need to check those ingredients as some will potentially be causing you harm. Ones to be aware of are:

1. Aluminium.
2. Polyethylene glycol.
3. Parabens (Butyl, Ethyl, Methyl, Propyl).
4. Diethanolamine (DEA), Monoethanolamide (MEA) and Triethanolamine (TEA).
5. Mineral oil.
6. Synthetic fragrances.
7. Triclosan.
8. Propylene Glycol (PG).
9. DMDM Hydantoin.

Again, I go into more detail on the above as it's a minefield, with a lot more than just what's listed to avoid, on my website:

www.thelongevityclinic.co.uk.

Environment

In the next section, we cover work dangers in more detail, however, if you live on a busy road, near or next to transport hubs such as train stations and airports or factories pumping out smog and other toxins, then I would simply move. I am not going to mince my words here and do some gradual phasing out of this problem, you simply need to move, as the damage this pollution is doing to you is incredibly dangerous.

This is simply not up for negotiation, if you are serious about living longer.

This leads me nicely on to the next thing, I still can't believe when buying a new house, people completely ignore electricity lines! There is a lot of research that indicates there are no health risks from ELF (extremely low frequency) radiation, the type that's emitted from power lines.

However, sometimes I feel you need to apply some common sense, as research papers can have numerous backers with large amounts of self-interest and power. Again, remember the tobacco companies claiming smoking was safe, with research based evidence, in fact sugar groups have been known to "pay" researchers to help their side!

I have very little evidence to back this up and it's up to you, what you believe, however, I practice what I preach and simply would not be living near electricity lines or any form of power generating station. The simple reason being, that it sounds absolutely incredible when you are near them, combined with that level of power, we are yet to find out what damage it can do long term with credible independent studies, so why take the chance?

Having neighbours who regularly create excessive noise that continuously irritates you (suppose it's different if it's your favourite band played loudly), needs to be rectified, as this will create a chronic form of stress and annoyance, which really is not good for your health.

You have a few options:

- Speak nicely to them.
- If they don't agree, accept this if you want to continue living where you live and forget about it.
- Speak with the council.
- If that can't be rectified and it annoys you that badly, simply move.

Work

Ever heard of the phrase "sick building syndrome"? Well it's true that some offices and work environments can quite literally be killing you, which I get since for some people they are just "dying to get to work"!

65

There are many causes at work (pun intended!), that will damage your health, though a lot can be improved or removed, by simply opening a window and letting that amazingly fresh and healthy air in, however the problem lies in: can you actually open an office window ten stories up? Of course not!

Also, if you are a in building that does have windows, I am sure you are fully aware of the arguments that soon start, by the influx of this newfound fresh yet cold air, with Trevor complaining about his papers flying everywhere, while Tracey moaning that she's cold! You have now opened a can of wormdows…

Never mind the noise from the traffic going past outside and that's before we get to the real evil, the pollution from a congested city…

Sealing a building from outside fresh air, creates an environment whereby every breath you take, is raising the carbon monoxide levels in the building. If there are enough of you, with no ventilation, this will cause you drowsiness and headaches, the exact opposite to what you want from your staff.

Now I can hear a few of you out there saying, well my brand spanking new office has air conditioning, so there! And yes, on that 30°C degree summer day, you are very much the envy of other office workers (particularly public sector workers, who I pity in their old sweltering outdated offices, with no air con) however where does this air-conditioned air come from?

Well, it's sucked in from outside, then circulated around your office. Being an office, you are most likely in a city/town centre or a business park, which of course are nearly always next to a, wait for it… motorway (it's a selling point!). So, you are having all this highly toxic air, sucked into your building and delivered right to your nostrils!

If your air con has filters, then you are fine but guess what, these systems are more expensive and what do companies like to do... keep costs down!

It gets worse, as the US Environmental Protection Agency (EPA) has stated that air pollution is often two to five times greater inside than outdoors, and at its most extreme can be one hundred times worse than outside!

A toxin-free alternative that would benefit everyone in the workspace is to add some plants to help purify the air naturally. Snake Plants, Spider Plants and Aloe Vera are notoriously good at this and along with improving the air quality for everyone, they also add a sense of tranquillity and help relieve stress too. Cost-effective and nice to look at, it's a win-win all round.

We've already covered things such as cleaning products and building materials in the home section of this chapter, but the same principle replicates itself in the workplace. As a quick recap, don't forget about the volatile organic compounds from paints, carpets and furniture used in the building. These escape into the air that you breathe, for sadly quite a number of years after being fitted, in what's known as "off gassing".

The main issue you have here, is that once you are aware of the issues you have at home, you have the power to be able to change them, whereas in your workplace, you often have little control over these. Unless you are a director, own the business or make everyone else aware, getting everyone on board, to force through change, which is very ironic for a capitalist as I actually sounded quite socialist here!

Now this part is not relevant for everyone but some of you reading this will have dangerous jobs. I will cover shift working on the sleep section however if you work on shifts, STOP NOW.

It is KILLING YOU. It's that simple, just STOP!!!!

Certain jobs put you in dangerous work environments, though they may not cause disease, they do put you at high risk of death! Why do something that can kill you, when you can do something far more enjoyable that doesn't kill you?

There are other jobs, that although there is no risk, will actually slowly kill you, by what you come into contact with, day to day. This could be chemicals or toxins in the air, jobs such as:

- Rubber manufacturing.
- Mining.
- Farming (unless an organic farm).
- Hairdressers.
- Metal work.
- Nail technicians.
- Decorators.
- Plastic Manufacturing.
- Stressful jobs in general.

Finally, building on the last point, certain jobs just seem to attract stress, and this is certainly a great way to die young, and never even get the chance to stink of piss at 90!

Things like being a solicitor, journalist, paramedic etc are difficult and I am sure for a lot of you, your jobs could easily be added to that list.

It's not just the type of job you do that can be stressful, it can also be your work environment. If you have a really horrible boss or colleagues and dread going into work each day, to have to continuously confront these toxic people, it can really play havoc on your mental wellbeing.

There are multiple factors that cause your work environment to be toxic to your health, though simply being aware of this, is a huge leap forward and once you make yourself aware of these factors, you can then put plans in place to address this. Whether that's having a word with a few people or even getting a new job, always remember your life depends on it!

Plus, on a lighter note, I suppose it could be worse, you could work in one of those Chinese nail bars! Where I feel like I am being gassed, just by walking past those places and that's with the door shut!

<u>Orally</u>

Processed food e.g. the meals you have to prick the top with a fork and ping it in the microwave, in order to eat, are seriously bad for you. They have high level of chemicals/preservatives (toxins), often low in fibre, high in sugar and severely lack nutrients, therefore they are dead calories. And to just add insult to injury, they come stored in a BPA toxic container! And then, when that's heated up, leaches these harmful toxins into your food. That before we even mention emulsifiers!

A recent study of 45,000 people in France over a seven year (yes seven years) period, showed that for every 10% increase in the amount of processed food consumed. It was associated with a 14% greater risk of death from ANY cause. Do I need to say anymore? So, stop forking your food!

As mentioned above, be very careful with what passes your lips (yes girls, often wise to do to a toxicity test on your new boyfriend!) that has been stored in a plastic container due to the toxicity of BPAs. Water is a good example, something that is good for you, yet somehow man has managed to tinker with, and the result is an end product, not so good for you. Which is why it's always best to keep things as natural and basic as possible.

While on the topic of water, your tap water has many harmful chemicals and heavy metals lurking around yet invisible to the human eye, so for this reason, you need to be religiously filtering your water.

The great thing is, it is actually really simple to do and very cheap. I have been using a Wellness Carafe for the last 8 years, which is simple and effective to use, which I keep in the fridge. This filters out fungus, bacteria, parasites, lead, mercury, chromium while also increases dissolved oxygen in my water.

In my next book, I dedicate a whole chapter to water, as it's a magical liquid and a few paragraphs in this book, just doesn't do it justice!

I don't even need to cover cigarettes, we all know what they do, and we all know nicotine is one of the most, if not the most, addictive substance in the world. It's hard to give up, though possible, as millions do it every year, I still have the odd cigarette drunk and hate to say, it does feel amazing after a few pints! That being said, boy don't I pay for it the next day! A worse hangover, bad throat, while my next run is super tough to say the least!

Again, I don't want to cover well-trodden ground by people with far more expertise and experience on these subjects than me, however when you start to understand the body more, this helps with cutting back on the booze. When you know what it does to you, it really makes you take a second thought and go should I really have that next drink!

Meditating has also worked really well for me, whereby I now don't feel the need to keep drinking, until either I've ran out of money or can no longer stand! It's really helped in allowing me to have just a couple, then call it a night earlier, with more money left in my pocket!

What I've learnt with regards to myself over the last five years is my hangovers are becoming deadly, as in lasting for up to five days in some instances, the reason being alcohol destroys production of the hormones that make you feel great and give you your 'get up and go'. Not only this, it fucks with the quality of your sleep. So, add the two together and you have super shit hormone production.

This is TERRIBLE for your moods and productivity.

I've found CBD oil has helped with this, as I can now muster motivation the next day after a late one. I also increase my Omega 3, Milk Thistle and B vitamins post drinking along with 4 charcoal tablets before and after drinking, much to the amusement of my friends!

Ironically it was my desire to still drink, yet not age and destroy my body, that got me into longevity in the first place. I thought if I could overcompensate in other areas of my life, this will counteract the booze. However, the more I learn, the less often I am drinking.

Always remember the old saying *"one's too many, three's not enough"*

The best way to stop people with bad addictions/habits, is to find something more enjoyable to do instead. So, your first point of call would be to think of something amazing, that you would love to do regularly, then simply go and do it! Also, the less free time you have, the less time you have to drink...

Sex is a good one, as most people enjoy this activity, so you can replace a booze addiction with a sex addition and as long as you wrap up safely, you have now given yourself a physically exerting hobby, so congratulations, just don't tell the wife...

Now on to food, if something has a label on it, don't eat it. This is a very good way to live your life!

Ideally no meals should require you to fork them hard, however the odd fork every now and then, isn't going to be the end of the world! It's also not as simple as just removing microwave meals, as foods like crisps, sausages, cakes, biscuits, breakfast cereals, pies, softs drinks etc., all fall into the processed food family.

The reason these foods are bad for us nutritionally are covered in more depth, in my next book in this series however in a nutshell, generally they contain high sugar, high carbs and low fibre.

This chapter is concerned with toxins and the biggies are:

1. **Bisphenol-A.** You're thinking never heard of it! Well, I bet you have. As they are widely known as BPAs, a chemical found in plastic, that leaches into the liquid or food that it is supposedly 'keeping safe' and storing! A huge example of this is plastic water bottles, I always have my water in glass to stop these dangerous compounds, from contaminating my body!

   BPA mimics oestrogen, by binding to the receptor sites meant for the hormone, which can disrupt normal hormone function. This is not the only hormone it's been thought to do this to, as thyroid hormone production, also suffers from the same process. In addition, high BPA levels have been associated with diabetes and infertility.

2. **Mercury.** Did you know that seafood is the biggest source of mercury in the human body! So ironically, what you thought was a healthy fish meal, has actually polluted you with a high-level toxin.

   Now I am sure you know that fish aren't made from mercury, it's more a case of the toxic waters they inhabit, being highly polluted by humans, with the mercury moving up the food chain, how ironic!

   Mercury is a serious toxin, in fact it's a neurotoxin, which damages your brain and nerves.

   Tuna is a mixed bag, as some brands especially canned varieties, can be highly contaminated, whereas anything caught far away from industrialised areas e.g. Alaska and stored in glass, are a lot better for you.

   However, there are certain fish types that are a complete NO these being Swordfish and King Mackerel.

3. **Vegetable & Seed Oils.** Vegetable oils bring no value to the table (get it!), as they contain no beneficial nutrients i.e. they are merely empty calories, while sadly being highly processed.

    They are high in polyunsaturated omega-6 fats which we do need, however not to this level! As we need to keep the balance of omega-6 and omega-3 fats, to around parity i.e. one-to-one and certainly not the six, eight or even 10 times, that the modern western diet exposes us to! High consumption of omega-6 linoleic acid can increase inflammation. This is very bad!

    This is all before we even come to what happens when we cook with vegetable oil and increase its temperature. They then release free radicals, that play absolute havoc with our body. Simply switch your vegetable oil for a spoonful of coconut oil, toxin-free and a great all-rounder to have in the house. From substituting cooking oil, mouthwash, even hair and body moisturiser, there's nothing this stuff can't do!

4. **Trans Fats.** These are the worst fats you could possibly consume! Due to the way they are made, by pumping hydrogen into unsaturated oils to turn the fat solid. Our bodies don't recognise trans fats, so therefore we can't process them in the same way as natural fats. The result is that sadly, trans fats cause inflammation.

    Inflammation is quite literally a secret assassin to mankind!

5. **PAHs (Polycyclic Aromatic Hydrocarbons).** Are toxic by-products from cooking red meat, when cooked at high temperatures on a grill. The fat drips onto hot cooking surfaces, producing PAHs that then seep back into the meat. Incomplete burning of charcoal can also cause PAHs, which have links to increased rates of prostate, colon and breast cancer.

If you can, it's best to use other means of cooking, however by minimising smoke and quickly removing any drippings will improve the level of PAHs produced.

6. **MSGs (monosodium glutamate).** Famously used in Chinese food (which is one good reason to throw that Chinese takeaway flyer in the bin, NOW!) however also very widespread in the processed food industry. It's a flavour enhancer and found in things like salad dressing, soups and frozen food but it's easy to spot just look on the label!

Summary

In line with the ethos of this workbook, I want you to actually do and action what's talked about here. This is why I have kept things as simple as possible, whilst also giving you enough of a reason "why". However, if any particular issue or toxin really took your fancy and you would love to learn more about it, then please visit my website:

www.thelongevityclinic.co.uk

where I go into a lot more detail about many of these issues outlined in this chapter.

This helps keep things straight to the point. Allowing you to action easily. Then when ready, you can go into more detail if that's something that you want to do. If you don't, it doesn't really matter as the main thing is that you are actioning everything in this book!

REMOVE - HEAT

Being super hot can kill you! Yes, hot people really die sooner AND have more health issues…

It's something that first was brought to my attention in 2017, having decided to start offering cryotherapy chambers for The Skin Repair Group, I embarked on the necessary due diligence. I was overwhelmed with all the health benefits, and it dawned on me, if cold is so good, then is heat bad for us?

This was further supported by my own dating experience, women that had serious health problems, tended to be very hot. Yes, they were good looking however, they were also like radiators to lie next to.

So why is heat bad for us? The obvious starting point, dare I say it, needs to be the news headlines. When we have a heatwave (as we have recently in August 2022), we see an increased number of deaths in the vulnerable categories such as the elderly and very young.

On a day to day level we notice that we don't sleep well in the sweltering heat and the impact on us mentally and physically the next day.

The resultant effects, from the heat exhaustion include dehydration, headaches, heavy sweating (think sticky uncomfortable skin), cramps, feeling sick, weak pulse and lack of motivation/tiredness (this aspect affects me the most as I struggle to get much done).

This excess heat is obviously not good for us.

It's worth pointing out, that numerous studies have shown how much slower you will perform, plus how less accurate you are, when it comes to any form of cognitive testing after being exposed to prolonged high temperatures e.g. heatwaves.

We've already covered pollution under toxins, however, it's worth noting how higher temperatures, increase the rate that pollutants react with atmospheric gases, to form ozone pollution.

This is where things get crazy, as a study in 2008 showed that for every degree increase in temperature, ozone pollution will kill an additional 22,000 people worldwide, due to respiratory illnesses.

It's not just outside heat that's killing people and making their lives a misery, your daily body temperature is as well. Inflammation is at the route of nearly all diseases that kill us (except for accidents). Inflammation by its very nature is heat, so for a lot of people who are hot, it will be due to increased levels of inflammation in their bodies.

Interestingly hot people will often have the following issues:

1. Taking medication, which further increases their temperature.
2. Hyperthyroidism.
3. Stress & Anxiety.
4. Multiple Sclerosis.
5. Fibromyalgia.
6. Diabetes.
7. Anhidrosis.
8. PMS.

9. Menopause.

10. Arthritis (this is why the joints radiate such heat).

A lot of the above are inflammatory issues.

Due to this, I do everything in my power to avoid extreme heat, ruthlessly pursuing a cool environment. One of the things I actively do at home is having an air conditioning unit in the bedroom. This is an absolute game changer, as I can now sleep during those rare but awful heatwaves, when the whole country is not sleeping, I am wrapped up in a blanket fasto…

That being said, short exposure to heat, like in a sauna or steam room is good for you, you don't need to stop these, it's the prolonged exposure to high temperatures, that you need to avoid.

Finally, it's up to you, are you going to be a sweaty betty or a cool cucumber…

How Hot Are You? Your Heat Checklist...

1. Do you wake up in the middle of the night hot regularly, even during winter months?

    ....

    ....

    ....

2. Do you ever break out in hot sweats/flushes randomly during the day?

    ....

    ....

    ....

3. Do partners ever comment, you are like a permanent radiator when in bed together?

    ....

    ....

    ....

4. Do any parts of your body often feel particularly hot e.g. stomach, back, joints?

    ....

    ....

    ....

5. Is most of your life felt feeling hot?

    ....

    ....

    ....

6. Describe how you feel on very hot days ie over 25C/77F?

    ....

    ....

    ....

7. How is this different to those around you?

    ....

    ....

    ....

Your Personal Notes

Time to Review Your Answers & Your Action Plan...

We've all heard the stories of those crazy old people who swim in near freezing lakes in winter yet live forever and NEVER get a cold. And what about those nutters, who have a cold shower every morning to "wake them up"?

Below are the key reasons, why you should also regularly be getting cold as well, followed by how best to do this:

1. **You Feel Amazing** - I just love getting cold for short periods of time, as I feel revitalised for some time afterwards, so regardless of all reasons below, it's worth doing just for this.

    The cold activates your endorphins, and it's these chemicals that make us feel good. The cold water acts as a "system reboot", as I like to call it. Sending many electrical signals to your brain, which account for a lot of the positive aspects listed here.

2. **It Reduces Stress** - By regularly getting cold, you are putting both your mind and body through a small level of stress, which long term, toughens you up the more you do it. Your nervous system slowly gets used to this regular, yet minor onslaught on your body, helping to keep you a lot calmer and more importantly, NOT stressed!

3. **Improves Your Circulation** - There are two sides to this, and as most people won't be going down to cryotherapy temperatures of -130°C, I shall explain the most likely situation. When your skin sensors detect the cold (though not life-threatening levels of cold), they send blood to the surface/extremities i.e. hands and feet, which helps flush your veins, arteries and capillaries., in turn strengthening them.

4. **Boosts Your Immune System** - In a nutshell, it boosts your white blood cell count, which is very good for you and the more often you

get cold, the better your body gets at activating its natural defences! Also, the shock of cold water stimulates leukocytes production, which help fight infections in your body. Though not proven yet it's likely related to an increase in your metabolic rate, which in turn stimulates your immune systems response.

5. **Improved Alertness** - The reason I have a cold showerearly on in the day after I've exercised, is that it wakes you up! This level of stimulation provides you with great levels of alertness, plus deeper breathing helps you to remove CO_2 from your body.

6. **Increased Willpower** - I'd like this to be easy, however, let's cut to the chase, it's not. Some mornings I think to myself, *oh do I have to...?* But then I am very glad I did afterwards. I find once you are in, it gets better very quickly (thankfully!), it's just that initial few seconds. You can further make this easier for yourself, by taking deep breathes, the moment the cold water hits you for the first time, this makes a big difference.

   By getting cold regularly, you are strengthening your willpower which then, obviously carries over into other areas of your life.

7. **Burn More Calories** - Exposure to cold in general (I'm sure most of you have heard the story about burning more calories having an iced water, than a room temperature water) helps you burn more calories. We've mentioned above how it increases the metabolic rate, which of course is amazing, it also stimulates the production of brown fat which in turn generates energy by burning calories.

8. **You Glow** - This is down to a previous mentioned benefit, improvement in your circulation, which in turn means you have an inner radiance, just like after exercising. I also find it tightens my skin, giving me a more youthful appearance!

REMOVE - CALORIES 8

For a long time, in fact probably over 20 years ago, I thought that surely the more we eat, the more we are using up our bodies. I used to relate it to 'putting mileage on the clock', using the car analogy, that the more we eat, the more we wear ourselves out and that our body has only so much capacity it can process, before we die.

Now I am not sure about the latter part, that we only have so much we can eat/process before we die, though surely there has to be a limit, as our bodies (yet) just can't go on forever. Plus, isn't it coincidental that all the centenarians are slim? Makes you think, although a fair few of them swear by a shot of whiskey too!

Fast forward 15 years and I started looking into fasting a lot more. I have never eaten huge amounts; however, the scientific evidence is completely overwhelming, that this really is the key to adding at least 10 years to your life...

Now I bet some of you will be thinking, this bastard wants to starve me, well he can piss off...

Well, would you like the good news? Of course you do - it's thankfully very simple to do.

My form of fasting is 4 to 6 days a week. I am not precious about it having to be exactly 6 days, as if I am away from home or socialising, I will throw aspects completely out of the window. I have looked a bit anal at some events in the past which is not good the first time you meet people by declining to eat most of what's on offer as you can come across picky, so now I just eat it. I do, however, notice the deterioration in my mood, energy and overall feeling. Which just serves as a great reminder, of the massive, short term benefits of fasting, even though the ultimate motivation for me, is many, many decades away.

I fast for approximately 23 hours daily, this means I have one meal a day at 1pm.

Now you don't have to skip two meals a day like me, but just skipping one meal a day is amazing and a huge game changer. I am also trialling at present 20 hours of fasting, with a four hour window of eating between 2pm and 6pm, the '*20/4 Fasting Plan*'.

It's also worth noting that my beloved mother, my favourite person in the world, is fat and when I say fat, I am not joking, she is grossly overweight. As a result, over the last fifteen to twenty years of her life, sadly she has had constant health problems

She is on painkillers, due to the intense pain in her knees, brought on by her excessive weight and lack of movement over the years. She can barely walk due to the pain, then if that wasn't bad enough, she now has dementia and very sadly is due to go in a home soon, where she will ultimately die in a few years. It's very heartbreaking to watch the decline, of such a fun, outgoing lady to this child like state, all based on a few lifestyle choices, made a few decades back.

All this has come about from her stuffing her face over the years, with little regard for her health. Please don't make the same mistake as her, otherwise you will spend the last decade or two of your life, like she has, in pain and going nutty!

Before we put a plan together for you, let's look at the benefits and then do a quick consultation together on your eating habits.

Benefits of Fasting

1. You will live longer (get to attend your great grandkid's wedding).
2. More consistent moods (stop falling out with colleagues before/after lunch).
3. More energy (get more stuff done).
4. A healthier body (think amazing abs).
5. Better sleep (better moods the next day).
6. Better concentration levels (better quality of work).

I like to keep things simple, otherwise the more I complicate things, the less likely you are to action what's in this workbook. One of the key ways that fasting is life changing, is it reduces your insulin levels in the blood, which is key for increasing fat burning.

The fat burning doesn't stop there either, as we also produce more growth hormones when fasting, which can increase many times over (think three to five fold, not just 30% extra!). These are great for fat burning and not so surprisingly given their name... muscle building as well!

Now who doesn't want to have less fat and bigger muscles?

Anyone here got diabetes? Well, the good news keeps coming! You guessed it. Fasting reduces your insulin resistance, by reducing your blood sugar levels. One of the most important things we need to do, is to lower blood sugar levels as that stops/reduces any sort of chronic disease. *Note- I am not a medical professional, please do speak to your GP if you have any serious medical condition before changing your diet.*

While I am at it, fasting also helps with oxidative stress, the whole thing where crazy molecules called free radicals, go off and cause mayhem in your body. Think of it as a naughty mischievous child, causing problems when it's not welcome!

One last point is that fasting, really helps with cell waste removal, in a process called autophagy. Autophagy eliminates the dead cells out of your body, that we really don't want anymore! These waste products can in fact lead to health issues if we allow them to be stored up over time. So, it's key, we remove these dysfunctional proteins from our body.

Though there are a lot of other benefits from fasting, this is a beginner's guide to living longer, so I will stop here as we have a fact find for you to do now...

How GREEDY Are You? Your Eating Checklist...

1. How often do you eat a day?

   ....

   ....

   ....

2. What times of the day do you eat?

   ....

   ....

   ....

3. Do you keep your eating times consistent?

   ....

   ....

   ....

4. Do you eat after 7pm? If so, how many times a week?

   ....

   ....

   ....

5. After meals do you feel full, bloated or can't move and just want to sit on the sofa?

....

....

....

6. How many courses do you have with each meal?

....

....

....

How often do you eat a day?

By just reducing what we eat, by around 30% to 40%, can make us live potentially **10% or eight years longer.** This really is an easy thing to do, it just means skipping one meal a day. I have found, though I love breakie, that breakfast is the easiest to skip.

It's also quite handy as well, as it saves you time in the morning, you are no longer preparing and cooking food, having to eat the food and then tidy up after yourself. This can easily add up to an extra half an hour, added back into your life, every single day. Put another way, this is 14 hours a month, and with this amount of extra time, who needs to live longer!

In order to help me through the day I have the amazing Bullet Proof Coffees. These are simply immense, they really keep you fuelled up for the day ahead while also being extremely good for you. They include MCT C8 oil and all the vitamins in organic grass-fed ghee such as Vitamins K, E & A, Omega 3 & 9, Conjugated Linoleic Acid (CLA) plus high quality saturated fat.

For more information on Bullet Proof Coffees, I have written an article on www.thelongevityclinic.co.uk website for those who want to pursue this further.

I would start off just skipping one meal to begin with and if you feel up for taking things to the next level, try as I do, by skipping lunch some days as well…

If this doesn't work for you, then you can always just go back to skipping breakie during the week and remember you don't need to be doing this every day, just weekdays is fine!

Do you keep your eating times consistent?

Your body likes consistent regular habits and patterns, whether this is going to sleep, waking up or eating. Try and keep the times you eat approximately the same every day, you will also get into a good habit for planning your day as well, though not the objective just a "Brucie Bonus"!

Do you eat after 7pm?

I eat most days at 2pm, this gives me plenty of time for my food to be well digested, by the time I go to bed around 10pm.

You need to ensure, as an absolute minimum, that you are leaving at least 3 hours, between your evening meal being devoured and your bedtime.

This is key for a number of reasons, the most important being, that you don't want your body having to process food while you sleep, sleep time as we cover in the sleep chapter, is for the body and mind to reset, repair, clear out all the toxins and grow!

After meals do you feel really full, bloated or can't move and just want to sit on the sofa?

You are eating too much. Plain and simple. Reduce your portion size.

If you enjoy feeling stuffed and unable to move, carry on as you won't be lasting long on this planet!

How many courses do you have with each meal?

The whole, eating multiple courses at each mealtime, was created by profiteers! Restaurants wanting to sell you more, yet you don't need more.

A lot of the western world's common practices boil down to money and greed (no I am not a socialist and will reiterate again, I am in fact a capitalist).

Just because it's expected of us to eat more than one course, don't! You don't need it; we get a lot more fulfilment out of eating just one good meal.

IMPROVE...
WHAT'S NEW PUSSY CAT!

IMPROVE - SLEEP 9

Did You Wake Up Tired This Morning?

I realised a few years back, that it's not the quantity, its more the quality, of sleep that's key for us humans!

Sleep is THE MOST important thing and luckily one of the simplest things, you can do today to change your life. It will make you live longer, feel happier, look younger, allow you to get more work done AND better work done, plus reduce the frequency that you get ill.

Need any more persuasion? If so, don't bother reading this, as you obviously have more important things to worry about than being super healthy and living longer...

Having invested in a sleep monitor in 2018, I have observed my sleep for a long time now and have seen first-hand, how the below actions, have seen my deep sleep and REM improve and surpass three hours most nights. My next goal is, to regularly achieve three and a half hours deep sleep and REM. With the ultimate aim of four hours plus, deep sleep and REM, in a window of between seven and a half to eight and a half hours in bed.

I deliberately use the word regularly, as opposed to "every" night, as appreciate some nights you might be staying at a hotel and therefore away traveling, exposing yourself to numerous factors outside of your control, while the ones normally within your control are temporarily harder to adhere to.

Please note you are not hard if you go without sleep and brag about it, you are just a fucking idiot!

Before we go through what we can do to improve your sleep, let's do a quick fact find to establish your sleep patterns and habits.

Your Sleep Checklist

1. What time do you go to bed?

   ....

   ....

   ....

2. Do you wake up the same time every day?

   ....

   ....

   ....

3. Are you on electrical devices like phones and laptops in bed?

   ....

   ....

   ....

4. Do you get a good dose of natural light first thing in the morning?

   ....

   ....

   ....

5. Do you exercise daily?

....

....

....

6. If so, what time do you exercise?

....

....

....

7. What time is your last coffee of the day?

....

....

....

8. What time do you stop consuming liquids?

....

....

....

9. What time do you eat your last meal of the day?

....

....

....

10. Do you snack or consume any additional food later in the evening?

....

....

....

11. Do you drink alcohol most evenings?

....

....

....

12. Is your bedroom hot when you go to sleep?

....

....

....

13. Do you regularly have your windows open, so that you have fresh air in your bedroom?

....

....

....

14. Does light seep through your curtains or blinds (this can be through and/or around)

....

....

....

15. Do you work within 2 hours of bedtime?

....

....

....

16. Is your mind super active the moment you put your head on your pillow?

....

....

....

Your Personal Notes

How to Optimise Your Sleep Quality

Go to bed the same time every night

Not so important the actual time, as opposed to the time being the same every night. Different people, have different natural preferred sleeping habits, whereby they might be a night owl or an early bird. However, what they all have in common, is the need to have a consistent sleep pattern or circadian rhythm.

The same goes for what time you wake up, so keep it consistent.

I will add a slight caveat to that, if I wake some mornings and feel really tired, then I will simply go back to sleep, to ensure my body gets the rest it needs. I take the view, there is no point being up yet, if so tired, you can't or don't feel like doing much, so you may as well not do much while asleep!

However, there is another school of thought, who believe in sticking to the same time every day, regardless of how tired you are, in order to maintain your circadian rhythm. I also agree with this, though appreciate it is rather contradicting. There are pros and cons to both tactics, so I suggest you personally experiment and find out what works best for you.

Stop using electrical devices in bed or late at night

This is probably the biggest disruptor of the developed world's sleep! These devices do two really bad things when it comes to your sleep, the first, the blue light emitted from the bright screens stimulates you, therefore waking you up and it blocks the production of your sleep hormone, melatonin. This really is not good for you.

Secondly it keeps your mind active and stimulated, especially if you are checking emails or working late at night.

Get a good dose of natural light first thing in the morning

For the same reason as blue light is a sleep killer, a burst of natural sunlight first thing in the morning, is an amazing way to wake up and start the day. This helps stabilise your circadian rhythm, enabling a good night's sleep later.

Exercise helps you sleep

Exercising is one of the easiest and quickest ways to make you tired and in turn sleep much better. Quite simply the more energy you burn throughout the day, the more tired you will become at bedtime!

Make your last midday

The very nature of a stimulant is to make you more alert and provide you with more energy, which is the exact opposite to what one needs come bedtime! For this reason, by giving yourself many hours between stimulant consumption and bedtime, the majority of the effects from such stimulants as caffeine and energy drinks, will have diminished to very low levels (though still in your system in small doses), allowing you to sleep.

For this reason, ensure that no stimulants are consumed after 2pm and ideally if you can, midday!

Stop pissing at night

As men age, we seem to need more loo visits during the night, mainly due to an enlarged prostate. Now this is an instant sleep killer, being woken up from an amazing deep sleep to go to the loo.

It gets even worse if you then decide to put lights on to stop you stubbing your toe! Better is to familiarise yourself with the walk to your loo and take it slowly, so not to wake yourself up, being now able to leave your lights OFF!

I've found the best way to stop midnight loo breaks, is to stop consuming liquids after 5pm. I will still have the odd small drink, though it's very much kept to a bare minimum.

Stop eating late at night

Late night eating directs a large amount of your blood to your stomach, which in turn takes blood away from the rest of your body, where it is needed to repair, restore and cleanse your body of the daily stresses it endures.

By eating within three hours of sleeping, you are depriving the body of this amazing bodily function that optimises you, ready for the next day.

Though I am sure the exact amount of time varies between individuals, I have tested that two hours is not enough, while three hours is the absolute minimum, from my last meal to bedtime. With four hours being my typical daily habit, i.e. last meal 5pm and lights out 9.30pm.

Keeping meal times consistent, is also great for your circadian rhythm AND don't forget food consumed late at night, is more likely to be stored as fat, than used as energy!

Ensure your bedroom is cool for bed and not stuffy

By having a cool room to sleep in, you allow your body to become ready for sleep and in turn, this will allow falling asleep to be easier and the sleep you get to be deeper.

Conversely, it's hard to sleep in a hot bedroom, as we struggle to fall asleep and when we do, we are continuously waking up throughout the night. Just think back to those sticky hot summer heatwaves, when you just toss and turn all night sweating.

Great little tip for waking up when you want to, is the flip side of this. I use heat to wake me up (though not in summer as my heating is off), so by having my heating come on around 30 to 60 mins before I want to wake up, I naturally wake due to the increase in my body temperature. Which is the reverse of what you want when falling asleep!

Get black out curtains or blinds

This is a must and so easy to do. In fact, they are just £15/$20 on Amazon, they attach to the back of your curtains and can be fitted in about two minutes per curtain!

The difference is just immense, your room will now be much darker, which will help reduce the amount of external light stimulus that floods into your bedroom, keeping you awake at night.

You can take this one step further and remove the light at the edges, by taping the sides of your curtains down.

Calm that busy mind

I rarely worry, however I do have a busy mind, with lot of fun and interesting ideas continuously floating around, though interestingly they used to intensify, the moment I rested my head on my pillow! It was almost like my pillow was a brain stimulant! These thoughts tended to flow continuously and in turn would keep me up for an average of half an hour.

The best way I found, to stop this and calm my mind has been to stop work at 7pm, which gives me between two and three hours before bedtime. If I go past this time, I really notice the difference when my head hits the pillow.

Another tactic that I have developed, is to just stop your mind from thinking of any thoughts by saying SLEEP as I breathe out, then reminding yourself that most thoughts discussed with yourself now, will be forgotten come the morning, so you may as well not even bother wasting your time!

Drinking Alcohol

The nights that I have drank alcohol (more than just one or two pints), I sleep easily, though the quality is not great. I haven't yet got great data on my sleep when drinking, as I generally don't think to put my sleep monitor on, as typically have more fun things to do... like listen to The Beach Boys loudly and sing!

One HUGE aspect I have noticed, is that for at least one night after drinking, though more likely, it's two nights after drinking (i.e. three nights in total, if you include the night you drank), I now sleep a lot longer. Between nine and ten hours, my deep sleep and REM is actually less, which is crazy!! So am sleeping longer and getting less of what I really need i.e. the deep sleep and REM sleep, which is now reduced to under two hours.

Conclusion

My top five action points, therefore keeping things simple and concise, while increasing your likelihood of actioning are:

1. Consistency of sleep pattern i.e. go to bed at the same time every day and wake up at the same time every day. Be fucking ruthless on this, as I am!
2. Natural light and fresh air i.e. being outside in the morning.
3. Exercise, though better than not, if it's just walking for 20 mins or more, I have found this doesn't seem to tire me out enough to get a really deep sleep, it needs to be some form of "out of breath" exercise, to get the more, deep sleep we want.
4. Rest the mind before bed, an active mind has been my biggest issue for lying there for hours some nights, especially when I've got exciting plans or concerns on my mind.
5. Finally, wearing blue light filter glasses has allowed me to wake up a lot less during the night, I have two types - yellow glasses that are to

be worn in the afternoon and early evening, then red glasses (complete blockers) for the last hour or so at night, however these make the colours very limited when watching TV and quality of life pretty rubbish for the last 30-60 mins before bed.

IMPROVE - NUTRIENTS 10

gnore worrying about nutrients for the time being. We save this for the next book, however the reason this chapter is still here, is that I am making you aware of what nutrients you currently consume and that ultimately, it is very important. However, for the time being, ignore becoming obsessed with nutrients.

I would much rather, you simply remove the dangerous substances you are currently putting in your body. This is such a HUGE win, you deserve a gigantic pat on your back! It's for this reason, we can save nutrients for the intermediate book.

However, I can't resist and will say it again, the best advice anyone could ever give you on diet and nutrients is simply…

IF IT COMES IN A PACKET…
DON'T EAT IT!!!!!

IMPROVE - EXERCISE 11

Quite simply put, movement is key.

You want to be regularly moving, being static for long periods of time is just not good for you.

Exercise can take many forms and if you hate the gym - those classes where you have to wear bright coloured lycra or even outdoor sports - don't worry as there are easy solutions.

The key thing is that you move and move often. So, for those who don't like to exercise, start off with a regular walk every day, even if this is just for five or ten minutes, as long as it gets you in to the habit. Once you've done this for a few weeks, you can then look at increasing this to around twenty minutes, however, if you don't want to walk that long, then don't! The key thing is you are doing something, no matter how small.

I don't want to go into huge detail here as like everything with this workbook, the idea is to keep it simple so that you get on and just do it. I could talk about all sorts of HiiT, split sets etc. but this book isn't an exercise book, it's a book to help you live longer in the quickest and simplest way possible, without overcomplicating things.

Think to yourself what do you enjoy? Then start doing it. If you are not sure what you like, just keep trying different random types of exercises, until you do! I don't care what it is, as long as it is something.

Huge bonus point here… if what you do choose, happens to be outside, then you get the significant extra benefit of nature and her magical healing powers of fresh air and sunlight.

There are endless studies that list the ways that spending time in nature can improve our mental health and well being, and reduce stress levels. From walking with your dog(s) or family in the park, going for a lone walk in the forest or visiting the beach, spending time in nature is an instant stress reliever. If you have access to a green space at home, try and make it that bit greener and bring nature to your doorstop. Research has shown that people that regularly access nature live longer, so make use of what this planet bestows upon us and visit nature often.

I Like to Move It, Do You?

1. How often do you exercise a week?

   ....

   ....

   ....

2. What days do you exercise a week?

   ....

   ....

   ....

3. What exercise do you do?

   ....

   ....

   ....

4. Do you enjoy it and if so, why? If you don't, also why?

   ....

   ....

   ....

5.   What time do you exercise?

....

....

....

How often do you exercise a week?

Though you don't need to do formal exercise everyday, amazing though if you do! It's important that you are regularly moving throughout the day, every day.

What days do you exercise a week?

If you have set days you exercise, this is great, as you most likely have now formed a habit, whereby you will stick to this. If you haven't formed a habit yet, by exercising the same days, every week, this will soon form a great habit for life...

What exercise do you do? Do you enjoy it and if so, why? If you don't, why?

One of the key things about exercise is that you need to enjoy it! If you don't, try something else out and as previously mentioned, sex counts, so why not try your wife out for a change!

The reason enjoying exercise is key, is that we want you to stick at it, until the day you die! When you enjoy something, you are more likely to keep up with it.

Obviously, the reverse is true, if you hate road running (I have huge doubts over the benefits for those long distance runners, come their later years, as they will be needing new hips and knees) then sooner or later you will stop. Once you stop there is a big risk you will stop for some time, if not for good!

What time do you exercise?

It's been proven time and time again, the best time to exercise is first thing in the morning. Why? Well for me (and what the scientific studies also confirm) is that I know it's done, there is no, well I'll just finish what I am doing and do it later... well later often never comes! It's a great feeling knowing it's done and conversely, I don't have that nagging feeling on my mind throughout the day, that I've yet to exercise today.

Next there, is that amazing feeling you get after you exercise, now if this isn't a fantastic start to your day, then I don't know what is! It helps improve your mood, your focus and the quality of your work.

Then finally for you vain buggers… like me, you get to look wonderful, from that glowing, radiant skin you get, from all that blood pumping around your face, that makes you look a million dollars!

On the reverse side to all these positives, if you exercise late at night, you are releasing stress hormones into the blood, leaving you in a state of alert. However, if the only time you can exercise, is late at night, do it. Exercising is always better than not exercising, regardless of the time of day, it's just better earlier on in the day.

IMPROVE - INFRASTRUCTURE 12

This has to be the most disregarded and overlooked LONGEVITY aspect!!!

Before I reveal what it is, I pose a question to you... would you like to ache or be in agony every time you moved?

Would you like to struggle walking upstairs, tying your shoelaces or even simply getting out of bed in the morning at some point in your 60s, 70s, 80s or 90s?

If you don't look after your infrastructure, then this will certainly be the case.

I define your infrastructure as your skeletal structure, muscles, ligaments and joints.

These are so key to our mobility and without mobility, we are grumpy miserable buggers! Never mind not being able to do all the things you want.

We only get one body, so please treat it well. I've seen people treat a shitty new build house (plus it'll probably fall down after a few decades, if one of the big house builders have built it!) better than their bodies!

Ask yourself, what's the benefit of having a great mind and highly functioning organs, if your body's structure doesn't work and you are in pain when you move? This is what amazes me about a lot of the health, wellbeing and longevity advice around, it misses this key point.

Number one on the list, has to be stretching. This is key to keeping your body flexible as you age and stopping it from going stiff, yet this is so often overlooked. This is pure madness. I stretch (almost) everyday, though yes, I do forget sometimes, while other days I am out all day with a ram packed schedule of meetings.

Like all things in this workbook, the motivation for doing them and writing about them, is for you and I to live longer. However, what I find is that we get massive instant gratification as well from a lot of these things.

It's like sex. Why has nature made that feel so good for us? It's as nature wants us to do it and do it lots, so in turn, we produce lots more mini versions of ourselves, to continue populating this planet!

Straight after stretching, I have these amazing waves of release. I can feel the tension leaving my body and it feels amazing! After my daily lying down on my back for ten to twenty minutes with a book under by head, I can feel the tension leave my lower back. This also leads to a great upright stance and posture, which in turn makes me feel more confident. I strongly recommend you give it a go.

Though I appreciate this can't be done yourself, I really enjoy having a massage, during it I can feel the knots and tension being worked out of my body. Then afterwards when I sit in the car to drive home, I just feel so relaxed, with quite literally the weight of the world, lifted from my shoulders.

Bend it Like Beckham... How's Your Structure Today?

1.   Do any of your joints hurt? If so, which ones?

....

....

....

2.   How long have the joints hurt for?

....

....

....

3.   Do you have any stiff muscles?

....

....

....

4.   Which muscles are these and how long have you noticed this for?

....

....

....

5. Do you slouch when standing?

   ....

   ....

   ....

6. Do you slouch when sitting at your desk or driving your car?

   ....

   ....

   ....

7. How would you rate your posture, out of 10?

   ....

   ....

   ....

8. How supportive would you rate your bed, out of 10?

   ....

   ....

   ....

9. Do you stretch, and if so, how often?

....

....

....

10. What muscles do you stretch?

....

....

....

11. Do you have regular massages? If so, what muscles do you focus on?

....

....

....

12. Do you lie down on the floor for 10 to 20 minutes with a book under your head regularly?

....

....

....

13. Do you eat food high in collagen or take collagen supplements regularly?

....

....

....

Your Personal Notes

Limiting Joint Pain Now and in the Future!

Ironically, one of the best things you can do to reduce pain in your joints, even if you already have gotten to this point, is move. I'm hoping that you haven't gotten to this stage yet, but the advice still sticks, just move. Movement provides your joints with more lubrication, so joints can move more smoothly.

I've covered movement before in this this book and movement is so key to us living long, fulfilling and most importantly healthy lives, so please just move and move regularly!

This book is all about prevention rather than cure, yes, the very opposite to our healthcare systems in the west! So, continuing with the books theme, here are some of the things I do, which means you can as well, plus they are cheap and easy to do, to stop you from being a walking wreck in your 90s…

I don't run for long distances as just as food, we have a limit to how much our bodies can take (well, for the time being until genome and stem cell therapy become readily available to all). By pounding your knees, hips and ankles continuously, they are going to break down eventually. The same way that you rub a piece of wood with sandpaper, eventually it will wear away.

That being said, by having a great diet, running with great form, wearing supportive footwear and choosing your running surface carefully, you will greatly improve your joints for decades to come.

Keeping this theme and moving away from long distance running/endurance activities, if you choose low impact activities and you don't weigh a lot, this will also reduce the stress and strain on your joints, its basic gravity, allowing you to move freely for longer.

As I've said multiple times, this stuff is super simple, it just needs a little nudge in the right direction, which is this book's (and my) job!

You've probably (I hope) noticed by now, that inflammation seems to be a recurring theme with this whole living longer thing. Keeping inflammation under control now, will stop you aching and being stiff as you age (and as good as the latter maybe for an erection in your 90s, your knees certainly won't be thanking you for the stiffness!).

I remember as a child my father regularly eating vile smelling sardines, stinking the kitchen out, then lecturing me about how good these are for your joints. Obviously at the time I was just annoyed about the smell and completely ignored him, like a lot of teenage boys do to their parents at that age, however, the bugger was bloody right. The omega 3 in sardines and other fish sources such as salmon, mackerel etc plus avocados, nuts and supplements, reduce inflammation in our joints, as well as your blood, while also being amazing brain food!

Whilst on the topic of nutrients and supplements, collagen is an absolute wonder for your body. Most people who are familiar with collagen, most likely will have heard about it from the benefits it provides to your skin. However, you will be more thankful for what it does to your joints, than looking sparkling at 90!

Collagen is a glue (protein) that holds our body together. From around 20 years old, it decreases at the rate of around 1% per annum, so yes when you are 90 you have 70% less of the stuff! Not good.

However, we can replenish collagen through our diet as our bodies can make it from protein, vitamin C and copper. Great sources of collagen include chicken, bone broth, fish, egg whites and the form I take it in daily, grass fed bone broth powder.

By boosting our collagen, we are providing our cartilage with the resources to slow down the rate at which it thins. Think of cartilage as a lubricant, that allows our bones to move smoothly over and along the connecting bone e.g. your knees.

Limiting Stiff Muscles Now and in the Future?

You may laugh at this, but I genuinely believe if the UK government provided a quarterly massage (or even annually) to people, then the NHS bill would be greatly reduced, however they don't, so here we go…

I have been having sports massages for almost a decade, it started off as just once a month. It wasn't long before I realised, this would be a key part of my longevity habits and in fact needed to up my game. I now have them, not just every week, but in fact twice a week.

I used to live a three hour round trip from my masseuse, yet I would still be having them weekly. I would travel back home to Monmouthshire, every week, just to have a massage!

I have been to some therapists in the new places I have lived since moving away from my home city, who have been ok, while some that have been good, though none to the level of Marie. It's for that reason, it really is worth investing the travel time, so that my 90 year old body, is free from stiffness and pain…

I mention this, to make you aware that not all massage therapists are equal, you just *know*, if you are having a good massage, so please be *very* selective, of who you choose long term, as it's the difference between a retirement full of movement and activity or one full of pain, misery and suffering.

Also make sure it's a professional sport massage, as we want the deep tissue aspect and not one of the superficial relaxing Swedish types (and on that note, a happy ending massage doesn't count either!). It's the deep tissue stimulation that helps treat muscle pain and improve any stiffness you may be experiencing.

Every day that you are on the planet, you are exposing yourself to more factors than can cause muscle pain and stiffness. So think to yourself, what happens if I let these cumulatively build up over not just years, but decades? Think of it just like your "back" account, if you store up lots of tension and don't expend it, then you will have a big store of muscle tension and pain, but unlike a large "bank" account, this one is not desirable!

Luckily sports and deep tissue massages are one of the best ways to release this pain, pressure and stiffness. By having them regularly, you are keeping on top of this build up. If you don't, the restriction in muscle movement will start to cause secondary effects. Like the restricting joint movement, which in turn causes the corresponding and overcompensating act, on the opposing movement/side of your body. All in all, an escalating downward spiral...

However, this is not the only reason why I have regular deep tissue massages, by bringing this much blood to the muscles and surface of the skin, you bring oxygen and valuable nutrients to the area, further increasing the quality of your skin and making you look super young, when perhaps you are not!

Even more important than looking fabulously young (when you are not) is that you are removing toxins stored up in the muscles, the fact that the toxins chapter is by far the longest chapter by some considerable margin, speaks volumes, about the effect of toxins on the body.

It reduces that 'i' word *inflammation*! Anything that reduces that, is a winner in my eyes.

I say this in a complete non-sexual manner, as I believe for us humans, the physical touch provided by massage, is also amazing for us through the soothing and psychological benefits. Though I don't want to go into this, as it's not what the book is about, they should not be overlooked, especially for those lonely and for their resultant wellbeing.

If that wasn't enough, even for the hardest of hard nose sceptics, it simply feels amazing having a sports massage. The actual treatment itself, feels good, it's perfect for reducing stress levels and then finally, when you come away from your massage, you feel beautifully relaxed and calm.

And Stretch…

This is one of my favourite daily routines and it's important for you to do, yet the great thing is that it can be done in under five minutes. Yes, that's right, one of the most important daily things we can do for our body, can be done in just a few minutes. Perfect!

As this is so important, I make sure I do this first thing in the morning as part of my longevity routine for a number of reasons. First, it's done. Yes done, no excuses, no distractions. Off the 'to do' list for the day.

Second, it's a great way to start the day feeling loose and energised.

A few little tips when you do stretch, is please don't bounce as this can cause more damage than good. Also, ideally stretching your muscles when they are slightly warm as opposed to cold.

Stretching has so many benefits, I will try to keep this quick, they are as follows:

1. Most people think of stretching as a way to minimise the risk of injury and they are quite right, it is excellent for this and if we want to live *"stronger for longer"*, then avoiding injury is key to that!

2. Release of tension, I find when I've done a really good hamstring stretch, I can feel the pent-up tension in my lower back, just disappear which feels divine! Such a great relief.

3. Muscles for a lot of people, store bottled up stress and emotions (this is why deep tissue massages are amazing!), resulting in your muscles becoming tighter. However, the more you stretch, the less tense your muscles become.

4. Increases your blood supply, which means a better you! With your lovely blood, comes oxygen and nutrients that supply the muscles with exactly what they need!

5. Flexibility is the main reason I stretch, as I like the ease and freedom of my movement. The more you stretch, the more flexible you become and therefore less stiff and it gets easier the more you do it!

6. Tranquillity, by taking a few moments out of your day to focus on just stretching and not worry or think about day to day issues, you provide your mind with a mental break, feeling a lot calmer and relaxed.

7. Which leads me on to my final point, posture. If you have stiff and tight muscles, you won't be able to stand upright correctly. You will instead have short and tight muscles, literally pulling you back. By stretching regularly, you now release these tensions and lengthen the muscle, allowing you to have an amazing posture.

Why Lying Down Will Improve Your Posture...

As I've previously mentioned but not gone into detail about, is that one of the things that's helped me the most for both my posture and to relieve any tension in my lower back, has been to lie down on my back, on a firm floor, with a book under my head and legs out straight. I had been doing this for years when someone suggested this is the "Alexander Technique", however that practice has the knees raised up, though it is similar.

I do this with my legs stretched out, then throughout my session I will change the position of my legs, from close together/parallel, to wide apart and moving my feet inwards to varying degrees, all in order to change the release of tension from my lower back.

I do this for ten to twenty minutes, five to six days a week, however, to get you into the habit, begin with just five minutes. Five minutes is better than none and in time, like I have, you will feel the amazing benefits it has for your posture and the release of tension in your lower back, so you will happily build this up to 20 minutes before long.

IMPROVE - MIND 14

The mind is such an incredible piece of kit we have and yet it's so easy to instead use it to harm us and oddly it takes a lot more effort for us to benefit from its tremendous power…

I don't want us to get lost by going too much into PMA (that's positive mental attitude) type thinking, however, there are in fact a few key mindsets, that will help you live a lot longer. Before we get onto those, it's that time again to ask you a few questions…

1. Do you think you are old?

    ....

    ....

    ....

2. Do you often catch yourself saying things like "not at my age" or "you're past it" and any other type of self-depreciating humour?

    ....

    ....

    ....

3. Are you lucky?

    ....

    ....

    ....

4. Are you playful?

    ....

    ....

    ....

5. Do you laugh a lot?

    ....

    ....

    ....

6. On average throughout the day, are your thoughts mainly happy or angry, sad, resentful and full of rage?

    ....

    ....

    ....

Your Personal Notes

You Are What You Think You Are....

Henry Ford said, *"If you think you can do a thing or think you can't do a thing, you're right"*.

So, on that note from, in my opinion, one of the world's greatest men, it's worth considering that if you think you are young, then just by simply believing this, your body will start to look, act and behave, as if it is young. I truly believe this.

Now I appreciate there are limits, as if you are getting drunk every night, smoking forty fags a day and eating a KFC before bed, then no amount of great thinking will counter act the catastrophic damage you are doing to your body!

In my mind I am late twenties (my chronological age is very different to the age I feel) yet I turned forty just a few weeks ago. As I am writing this, I feel young, super healthy, fit, my body functions well in all its capacities and I feel amazing inside. I am writing this in the morning after exercising, stretching, dry brushing, meditating, lying on my back for twenty mins, a butter coffee, 1.5lt of water, a cold shower and my goals, gratitude and visualisations, so perhaps it's no surprise, as this is my daily morning routine.

By ignoring your chronological age and allowing yourself to be the age you feel, or not even having a set mental age, just rather that "you are young" or "you feel young", is an amazing mindset for you to have, if you want to be "stronger for longer".

Just because this is simple, please don't underestimate the powerful effect your brain has on your health.

So, if you ever catch yourself in the future, saying things like "not at my age" or "you're past it" and any other type of self-depreciating humour, STOP.

135

Make that the last time, those terrible words come out of your mouth, and in fact remove them from your own self talk/dialogue while you're at it!

Related to this theme is that those who think they are lucky, get less illnesses and live longer. Study after study show this. Optimistic people have a reduced risk of heart disease, cancer, strokes, general infections and are more likely to live past 85.

A study of over 70,000 people, measuring their level of optimism has even proved this, way past the obvious common-sense view, that this of course would be the case.

As I write this, the last two years have been a terrible year for me; a close family friend died, my mum's dementia rapidly declined and she went into a home, due to the pandemic one of my businesses ceased to make any sales for eight months, yet I feel very excited and optimistic for the future, even if at this moment a lot of shit has been thrown my way. There are a few things I do to maintain my level of optimism.

Every morning I close my eyes for a minute or two and think of the top five things I am grateful for. Some mornings they may even be the same things as the last few days or even things I have mentioned loads before, which is fine, as I am still very grateful for them. This works wonders for your mind and is simple. They don't have to be major things either.

I used to write them out however some days I couldn't be bothered and found the best way to increase my uptake of this amazing habit, was by making it as easy as possible to begin with. And there are not many things easier, than simply closing your eyes for a minute!

A very recent strategy I have adopted, actually, this started in lockdown, was when something bad happens to you rather than get angry just laugh, it's so simple and so effective.

The first time I started doing this, was when a coffee I was making didn't just spill on the floor but went absolutely bloody everywhere, and I mean everywhere! Places that you couldn't even believe were possible and the kitchen was an absolute bloody mess.

Yet, I just looked at it all and burst into laughter, as it was so funny how it could even have begun to cause so much mess and I asked myself *why am I laughing*? I should have been be pissed off, as now I had a lot of mess to clean up, yet I noticed how happy I felt…

I am not sure how this process came about, though I am very glad it did. With this new outlook when things go wrong, I found it changes your day for the better. It's not what happens to you but how you to choose to react to what happens to you. Always look for the positive in all things, no matter how bad and this will help you live longer…

You can either be a annoyed, or lucky that something so funny happened to you…

YOUR PERSONALISED
LONGEVITY PLAN...

SUMMARY 14

By simply having read this book, you have now already taken in a lot of new information, both medical facts and those proven by my own personal experiences. You are now aware of a world, that perhaps, you weren't previously aware of? The real learning, however, comes in actioning what you have learnt and making the contents of this book, daily and general life habits.

It's for this reason, that I have created the following "Longevity Action Plans" for you. I really want you to start experimenting with the spirit of this book, and if this means starting with small steps, then that's one step further to helping you live longer.

I will finish this book the way it was started, by simply reminding you of what, if you really had to pick, which I hate having to do, as there are so many factors (though this book is about keeping it simple for you), are the absolute winners to take your life to the next level.

Below are the **6 key things,** you need to to pay extra attention to, in order to live longer, not stink of piss at 90 and to STOP KILLING YOURSELF:

1. Sleep (number 1 for a reason!).
2. Sugar.
3. Stress.
4. Toxins.

5. Fasting.
6. Exercise.

My *only* objective from reading this workbook, is that you take "some" action. I would love it if you did it all, as you will live a much "stronger for longer" life, however even if you just do a few things, this is amazing and will change your life significantly for the better.

As my job is to help make living longer, as easy as possible for readers, I have created two "action plans" to help implement the information and advice within this workbook. The first, chapter fifteen, is 'the bare bones', giving gentle steps and habits to follow that will enhance your life, without requiring any major life changes. It is my hope that this method will add a minimum of five years to your lifespan.

The second, chapter sixteen, really is 'the start of something special'. In this chapter, I build on chapter fifteen with methods that can greatly maximise your life and I hope will add at least ten years to your lifespan. Please note that some aspects will be repeated, but this is to save readers from going between the two chapters. Both options have a simple-to-follow plan in place to ensure you get the most out of this workbook as possible.

For those that want that something extra for added longevity, please see my website for a whole range of longevity options from one-on-one coaching, courses, and more in-depth research and findings that I purposely didn't include in the workbook, to keep it simple and easy to use.

Like most things in life, longevity and living longer is more fun if done together, this could be with your wife or husband, setting your children up for a great and healthy life, or with your friends to help each other out and point each other in the right direction.

So, without further ado let's get you living longer…!

GIVE ME FIVE (YEARS)... THE BARE BONES WAY TO LIVE LONGER!

15

Remove...

1. **Remove Sugar**

   Soft/Soda Drinks - Stop drinking anything that fizzes! To begin with, if you do have the dying need to have a fizz in your liquids, then choose carbonated water as a temporary measure to transition you over from the dark side, however by going for still water long term, you are making it easier for you to consume higher levels of water, as the bubbles fill you up!

   Sweet Snacks - This is just crazy! Why not, while stuffing your face with a cream cake at 11am, shoot yourself up with some smack!

   Check the Label - Any food you buy, check the label. You can now also do this with restaurant food. Though you will be horrified, by just how much the big chains are putting in your food. Use the basis that 37g of sugar a day is the maximum you should be having I have a lot less, though it's a great starting point.

2. **Remove Stress**

   Exercise - One of the fastest ways to burn off anxiety and worry.

Get Outside - Fresh air and being out of the environment that caused your tension, try and spend at least fifteen minutes outside a day where possible. No phones or tech, just you, and nature, a great way to reduce daily stress.

2pm Stimulant Ban - Get all your stimulants done and dusted for the day by 2pm! This will help you sleep a lot easier and in turn, will make you less stressed, more focused, more energetic and more relaxed!

Stop Beeping - Turn off all notifications, from the toxic mobile communication device you have permanently attached to you! This means texts, WhatsApp, emails, social media, news feeds etc. This is not stopping you from using these things (well except for the news), it's all about checking them at set times of the day e.g. 11am, 2pm, 5pm and not letting them interrupt your concentration.

3. **Remove Toxins**

Problematic People - Whether this is family, friends, neighbours or work colleagues. If these people are causing you problems, which have been unable to be resolved by a good sit down and chat, then simply remove them from your environment. Sometimes this can mean moving or quitting a job, yes, it's scary but it's fucking worth it!

Busy Roads & Transport Hubs - Living in close proximity to these are toxic for your health. There is only one solution and that's to move. I appreciate this is not what you want to hear, however, if you are serious about living stronger for longer, then this is what you need to do.

Smoking - Start by saving smoking for the end of the day or when out socialising with friends, as your first step to giving up. You are not stopping yourself from smoking, simply just reducing how much you smoke. Even if this means you never actually stop smoking. If we have gotten your smoking down from twenty a day to two a day, then this is a fantastic result!

Alcohol - The quickest and most effective step here, is to simply remove alcohol from your home. Your will power is lowest at the end of the day, when you are tired. Now think, if you have to leave the house and get in a car to buy booze when tired, rather than simply pop into the kitchen and grab a beer from the fridge, it's most likely that you can't be arsed to do this!

4. **Remove Excessive Heat**

    Cold Shower - The last 30 seconds of every shower you have, just reduce the temperature to cool (not cold) for five days, then after five days of cool, reduce the temperature further to cold.

    Extremely Hot Environments - Remove yourself from any excessively hot environment you find yourself in, whether you are on holiday and spent too long in the 30°C sunlight, or you are in a building that for some reason is stupidly hot!

5. **Remove Calories**

    Skip Breakfast - This one is easy, for just three days each week, skip breakfast.

    Late Night Eating - Aim to eat around 16:00 to 18:00 every evening, however I appreciate with work/commuting this can't be possible if you want to eat with your family every evening, so aim for no later than 19:00. Ensuring you have a full three hours, between finishing your last meal of the day and sleep.

Stop Being a Slug - If you are bloated or sluggish after a meal, look to reduce your serving size until this is no longer a problem. Quick caveat, it might not just be the size of your serving, it could also be the low-quality food you are eating e.g. processed; incorporate more fresh vegetables in your diet.

Improve...

1. **Sleep**

    Consistency - Go to bed and wake up at the same time every day. This is one of the most important lessons to learn for a "stronger for longer" life.

    Eat Early - Ensure the last thing you eat is at least 3 hours before bedtime, ideally the earlier you can eat the better eg between 16:00 – 18:00.

    Blue Lights - Stop using mobile phones/tablets/laptops at least an hour before bedtime. Do not bring mobile phones/laptops into the bedroom, leave them downstairs or in your office to charge.

    Stimulants - Stop consuming caffeine, energy drinks or other stimulants after midday, if you really must, 2pm at the very latest.

    A Cool Bedroom - Will help you fall asleep quicker and give you a deeper sleep. Close your curtains on hot days, to stop direct sunlight heating up your bedroom throughout the day, open your windows to allow cool fresh air in, have fans and air conditioning units to keep your bedroom chilled at night.

    Calm Your Mind - A busy mind will stop you from sleeping. If your mind is that stressed or active, it could mean in worst cases, not actually getting any sleep at night.

Stop any activities that over stimulate your mind like work, horror/action movies, electrical devices, arguments or worries within two hours of sleep.

2. **Nutrients**

Packet Food - This is super simple, though appreciate more difficult to action at first, if it comes in a packet, don't eat it! Best way to get into this amazing habit, is to start on your next shop, remove one in three of the packet foods you would normally buy, you don't have to remove them all, just gradually over the next month, so you hardly notice they are gone.

3. **Exercise**

Move - Every day and preferably in the morning, do some form of movement for at least five minutes, whether a gentle walk, quick jog to the end of the road and back, press ups, just anything really, to gently get you into the daily morning habit of moving.

4. **Your Infrastructure**

Stretch - Three days a week stretch to begin with, then working up to Five days a week, once you are in the habit!

Stand up Straight - Just be conscious of your standing position throughout the day and realign yourself. The a few times a week, simply lie on your back, on a firm surface, with a book under your head.

Collagen - Start consuming foods with high levels of collagen in, such as chicken, eggs and arguably the best though least appealing, bone broth, of which I have no interest in making hence why I take powder supplements. Worth noting that the drink/sachet supplements are expensive and don't have that high level of collagen in generally I have found.

5. **Mind**

Start Thinking Young - By thinking in a youthful and young frame of mind, you will notice your body believing that you are younger than you actually are this in turn, will maintain your body in a more youthful manner, than if you keep reminding it that you are now old!

Gratitude - The happier you are, the happier the signals your brain sends to the rest of your body, and in return, the less toxicity and bad energy you then trap in your body.

To further make your life easier, I have also created a simplified version of the above, in a checklist format which is available to download at **www.thelongevityclinic.co.uk.**

16

GIVE ME TEN (YEARS)...
THE START OF SOMETHING GREAT!

Remove...

1. **Remove Sugar**

   Soft/Soda Drinks - Stop drinking anything that fizzes! To begin with, if you really have the dying need to have a fizz in your liquids, then choose carbonated water as a temporary measure, to transition you over. However, by going for still water long term, you are making it easier for you to consume higher levels of water, as the bubbles fill you up.

   Sugar in Tea/Coffee - Stop putting sugar in your drinks. To start this transition, begin with halving what you previously put in your drinks for a week or two. Then ultimately, slowly but surely, wean yourself off this silent assassin.

   After Dinner Deserts - Deserts should be treats for special occasions if you have them, limit them to weekends or parties.

   Sweet Snacks - This is just crazy. Why not, while stuffing your face with a cream cake at 11am, shoot yourself up with some smack!!

Check the Label - Any food you buy, check the label. You can now also do this with restaurant food. In fact, you will be horrified, by how much the big chains are putting in your food. Use the basis that 37g of sugar a day is the maximum you should be having, I have a lot less, though it's a good starting point for you.

2. **Remove Stress**

Exercise - One of the fastest ways to burn off anxiety and worry.

Get Outside - Fresh air and being out of the environment that caused your tension, try and spend at least fifteen minutes outside a day where possible. No phones or tech, just you, and nature, a great way to reduce daily stress.

Turn off News - For those worried about the world and their country, this is one of the worst things you can be consuming. Just turn it off. You will also be very grateful for the time you save!

2pm Stimulant Ban - Get all your stimulants done and dusted for the day by 2pm! This will help you sleep a lot easier, which in turn, will make you less stressed, more focused, more energetic and more relaxed!

Stop Beeping - Turn off all notifications, from the toxic mobile communication device you have permanently attached to you! This means texts, WhatsApp, emails, social media, news feeds etc. This is not stopping you using these things (well except for the news), it's simply all about checking them, at set times of the day e.g. 11am, 2pm, 5pm and not letting them interrupt your concentration.

3. **Remove Toxins**

Problematic People - Whether this is family, friends, neighbours or work colleagues. If these people are causing you enough problems, which you have been unable to resolve, by a good sit down and chat, then remove them from your environment. Sometimes this can mean moving or quitting a job, yes, it's scary but it's fucking worth it!

Electro & Magnetic Field Radiation - Don't sleep with your phone next to your head e.g. placed on your bedside cabinet. Try to not have your phone on you in person e.g. in your trouser pocket and keep it in your briefcase, turn off WI-FI at night, use cable headphones, so that your phone is not close to your brain when in use.

Chemicals & Your Skin - A lot of the "anti-aging & wellbeing" products we use to help clean us, look younger or make us smell nice, will contain chemicals you do not want. Luckily our skin won't absorb them all, though still check the labels for things such as parabens, sodium lauryl sulfate, BHT and synthetic fragrance. There are others, however this is a good starting point.

Your Drinking Water - There are so many harmful chemicals and heavy metals in tap water, that you really need to be filtering all your drinking water. It's really simple to do and very cheap. I have been using a Wellness Carafe for the last eight years which is simple and effective to use.

Aerosols - Allergies are aggravated by aerosols and for those of you without allergies, you are exposing yourself to headaches, breathing issues and skin reactions. So always opt for the non aerosol option e.g. roll on deodorants and hair gum/wax.

Busy Roads & Transport Hubs - Living in close proximity to these are toxic for your health. There is only one solution and that's to move. I appreciate this is not what you want to hear. If you are serious about living "stronger for longer", then this is what you need to do.

Polluting Factories & Chemical Plants - These places are putting a lot of shit in the air that you breathe, and you want to be as far as way as possible from this place!

Smoking - Start by saving smoking for the end of the day or when out socialising with friends, as your first step to giving up. Initially, you are not stopping yourself from smoking just limiting how much you smoke. Even if this means you actually never stop smoking, if we have gotten your smoking down from twenty a day to two a day, then this is a fantastic result!

Alcohol - The quickest and most effective step here, is to simply remove alcohol from your house. Your will power is lowest at the end of the day when you're tired. So, if you have to leave the house and get in the car, to actually buy booze, rather than pop into the kitchen and grab a beer from the fridge, you are much more likely to not drink! Easy...

Plastics & BPAs - Avoid storing food or drink in plastic containers and instead use glass. You can now get BPA free plastics, however it's just easier to switch to glass to avoid this issue completely as you never know what else is in the plastic.

4. **Remove Excessive Heat**

Cold Shower – For the last thirty seconds of every shower you have, just reduce the temperature to cool (not cold) for five days, then after five days of cool, reduce the temperature further to cold.

Extremely Hot Environments - Remove yourself from any excessively hot environment you find yourself in, whether you are on holiday and spent too long in the 30°C sunlight or are in a building that for some reason is stupidly hot!

5. **Remove Calories**

Skip Breakfast - This one is easy, for just three days each week, skip breakfast.

Late Night Eating - Aim to eat around 16:00 to 18:00 every evening, however, appreciate with work/commuting, this can't be possible if you want to eat with your family every evening, so aim for no later than 19:00. Ensuring you have a full three hours, between finishing your last meal of the day and sleep.

Stop Being a Slug - If you are bloated or sluggish after a meal, look to reduce your serving size until this is no longer a problem. Quick caveat, it might not just be the size of your serving, it could also be the low-quality food you are eating e.g. processed; incorporate more fresh vegetables in your diet.

Improve...

1. **Sleep**

Consistency - Go to bed and wake up at the same time every day. This is one of the most important lessons to learn, for a "stronger for longer" life.

Eat Early - Ensure the last thing you eat is at least three hours before bedtime, ideally the earlier you can eat, the better eg between 16:00 – 18:00.

Blue Lights - Stop using mobile phones/tablets/laptops at least an hour before bedtime. Do not bring mobile phones/laptops into the bedroom, leave them downstairs or in your office to charge.

Natural Light - As early as possible every morning get a hit of natural light to help wake you up and stabilise your circadian rhythm.

Exercise - Is one of the quickest and easiest ways to make you tired, in turn falling asleep quicker and giving you a deeper sleep.

Stimulants - Stop consuming caffeine, energy drinks or other stimulants after midday, if you really must 2pm at the very latest.

Late Night Liquids - Limit significant liquid intake after 5pm, as this is likely to wake you up during the night for a loo break, which breaks your deep sleep. You don't want to be lying awake at 3am unable to get back to sleep, do you?

A Cool Bedroom - Will help you fall asleep quicker and give you a deeper sleep. Close your curtains on hot days to stop direct sunlight heating up your bedroom throughout the day, open your windows to allow cool fresh air in, have fans and air conditioning units to keep your bedroom chilled at night.

Blackout Blinds - Don't let external light sources keep you stimulated and awake at night. Block them out with blackout curtain and blinds, as normal blinds and curtains still let through a lot of light, even when closed.

Calm Your Mind - A busy mind will stop you from sleeping. If your mind is that stressed or active, it could mean in worst cases, you not getting any sleep at night.

Stop any activities that over stimulate your mind like work, horror/action movies, electrical devices, arguments or worries, at least two hours before sleep.

Drinking Alcohol - Reduces the quality of your sleep after even just one or two drinks, for this reason you will wake up even with your typical eight hours sleep, feeling less alert, less active and less motivated than normal.

2. **Nutrients**

Packet Food - This is super simple, if it comes in a packet, don't eat it! Best way to get into this amazing habit, is on your next shop, remove one in three of the packet foods you would normally buy. You don't have to remove them all, just gradually over the next month, so you hardly notice they are gone.

3. **Exercise**

Move - Every day and preferably in the morning, do some form of movement for at least five minutes, whether a gentle walk, quick jog to the end of the road and back, press ups, just anything really, to gently get you into the daily morning habit of moving.

4. **Your Infrastructure**

Stretch – To begin with, stretch three days a week, then working up to five days a week, once you are in the habit!

Stand up Straight – Simply by just being conscious of your standing position throughout the day, you can then realign yourself. Then a few times a week, simply lie on your back, on a firm surface, with a book under your head for 10 minutes.

Low Impact - Any form of exercise that you feel could be damaging your joints, look into, as I've heard a hip replacement is excruciatingly fucking painful!

Collagen - Start consuming foods with high levels of collagen in or taking powder supplements. The drink/sachet supplements are expensive and don't have that high level of collagen in I've generally found.

Massages - Find a great sport massage therapist and go at least monthly, though ideally weekly.

5. **Mind**

Start Thinking Young - By thinking in a youthful and young frame of mind, you will notice your body believing that you are younger than you are. This will maintain your body in a more youthful manner, than if you keep reminding it, that you are old now!

Gratitude - The happier you are, the happier the signals your brain sends to the rest of your body and in return, the less toxicity and bad energy trapped in your body.

To further make your life easier, I have also created a simplified version of the above in a checklist format which is available to download at

www.thelongevityclinic.co.uk.

Finally....

If it's in your house or in close proximity to you, you have increased your chance of consuming something that's bad for you.

I remove all temptations from my surroundings e.g. I have no ice cream or alcohol in my house!

Remove from your life, all the things you know that are bad for you and you have then taken the simplest, and best steps, to living longer.

Thank You for Reading...

Have You Enjoyed This Book?

I really do hope so, and if you have, I would be genuinely grateful for your thoughts and feedback to help improve the book and help others decide, if this book is for them.

Please consider leaving a review on Amazon or your favourite store.

WOULD YOU LIKE ANY FURTHER HELP?

17

We have a very comprehensive central learning centre on my website, **The Longevity Clinic**, that cover my Longevity Model "RIO – Remove, Improve & Optimise". The link is below.

In addition to my RIO Model on my learning centre, I also have comprehensive articles and guides specific to sleep, energy and longevity machines.

My website or LinkedIn is the best way to get in touch with me, so please feel free to connect with me on LinkedIn or via the website, if there is any way I can help you further?

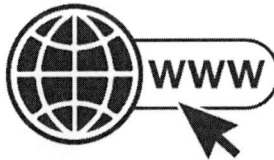

www.thelongevityclinic.co.uk

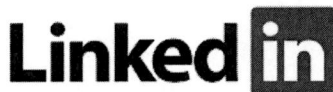

www.linkedin.com/in/ralphwmontague

Historically I have not liked anti-social media, another toxin on society's attention spans, while contributing to loneliness as people don't get the real face-to face-personal interaction that we all need as people.

However, it's not going away anytime soon. So, I can either get stuck in the past or join the party and bring something of value to the table with my sleep, energy and living longer findings.

So please feel free to watch my regular short videos on YouTube, and Instagram, where I update you on my latest articles published on Medium.com with my new perspectives to optimise you and your family.

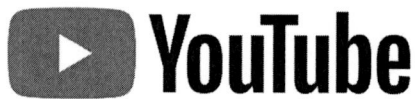

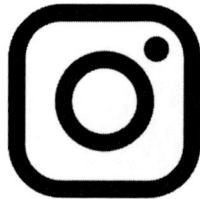

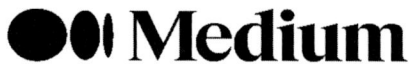

HOW RALPH CAN HELP YOU? 18

If you are looking at taking living longer seriously and making it a key part of your daily life, then there are a few ways Ralph can further help you, to achieve your longevity goals.

Depending on your learning style and preferences, Ralph can help you in the following ways:

1. **Longevity Coaching - Online Training Programs.**

    Sleep Mastery is a super easy to action, yet comprehensive coaching program for you to master the most important part of longevity…sleep!

    Energy Mastery will be released in 2023, which guides you how to have more energy, get more things done and live longer.

2. **Corporate Workshops – Onsite Training Programs.**

    If you would like your employees to perform at higher levels, make your business more profitable, all while feeling happier, then the Sleep Corporate Workshops can do this for you.

In addition to your workforce, if you would like a more personalised approach for board members and senior staff, this option is also available.

We also offer Energy Corporate Workshops for those that have first done the Sleep Corporate Workshops.

To find out more about the above, please visit the website www.thelongevityclinic.co.uk.

ABOUT THE AUTHOR
RALPH MONTAGUE

19

Having been raised in Monmouthshire, before leaving to study at Reading University, where Ralph studied for his Bachelor's in Investment Banking and Master's in Commercial Property, a career in stock broking was the intended path.

It wasn't long before the urge to do something in the anti-aging world took over his banking and property aspirations.

With Ralph's first anti-aging and aesthetic clinic in 2005, looking and being younger has always been key to Ralph's heart.

Ralph was the founder of The Skin Repair Clinic, a regional chain of aesthetic clinics and previously, a director of The Skin Repair Group, a provider of anti-aging and longevity devices such as cryotherapy and hyperbaric oxygen therapy.

He is a multi-author having written the UK's leading aesthetics business book, The Profitable Clinic. With more to come...

His passion for longevity evolved from the anti-aging industry he'd been so heavily involved in, which was the basis for The Longevity Clinic. As founding partner, the aim of The Longevity Clinic is to educate and guide people in the simplest way possible, on how not only can they increase the age at which they die but more importantly live a healthy and happy life, right until the end. With no chronic diseases pestering them for the last decade of their lives.

Ralph certainly practices what he preaches, having a Cryotherapy Chamber, Localised Cryotherapy Device, Hyperbaric Oxygen Chamber (HBOT), Oxygen Facial Device, a Skin Repair Pen (micro needling), Fat Freezing Machine, Red Light Therapy, HIFEM Accelerated Muscle Stimulation machine and his most recent addition Adaptive Oxygen Therapy machine (Intermittent Hypoxia), all at home for his personal use and he absolutely loves all these things, using them multiple times a week!

Though no saint, you will still see Ralph out and about getting drunk a few times a year. Plus, his weekly pizza or curry, though the McDonald's are now just for emergencies when out on the road, and that's the message he wants to spread, you don't have to be perfect and super anal all the time, just most of the time…

FURTHER READING & REFERENCES

20

For those who want to dig deeper and explore the themes covered in this book in greater depth, then below is a great starting point for you, they form part of my research, used to write this book, that back up my plans for a long and healthy life.

There is a very deliberate reason why I haven't included them in this book, as I don't want people to get lost in the science, so that they take action. The below add around an extra 100 pages which could overwhelm people and cause analysis paralysis!

The following topics are available to read (some have videos) on my website www.thelongevityclinic.co.uk, for you to make delving deeper as easy as possible for you.

1. The Best Beds in the World.
2. Cryotherapy Chambers.
3. Hyperbaric Oxygen Therapy Chambers.
4. Red Light Therapy.
5. Intermittent Hypoxia Therapy.
6. Botox.
7. Pesticides.
8. BPAs & Plastics.
9. Sweeteners.

10. Food Additives.

11. Skin Care Toxins (deodorants, cleaning, moisturisers).

12. WIFI & Mobile Phones.

13. Washing detergent.

14. Kitchen Cleaning Products.

15. Paint.

16. UV lights.

17. Foam Bedding.

18. Carpets & Curtains (VOCs)

19. Aerosols.

20. Tap Water Contaminants.

21. Lead Piping.

22. Fluoride.

23. Air Conditioning.

24. Burnt Foods.

25. MSGs (Mono sodium glutamate).

INDEX

A

adrenaline, *25*
Aerosols, *151*, 166
aesthetics business book, *7*
Air Conditioning, 166
Alcohol, *152*
allergies, *61*
Aluminum, *64*
Alzheimer's, *15*
American Heart Association, *19*
Anhidrosis, *76*
anti-ageing industry, *7*
arsenic, *56*
autophagy, *86*

B

Being contactable, 23
benefits, 59
Bisphenol-A, *72*
Blackout Blinds, 154
blood pumping, 116
blood sugar level, *85*
Blue Lights, 153
bodies healing mechanism, *16*
body, 70
bombardment, *24*
Boosts Your Immune System, 81
Botox, *36*
Botox., 165
BPAs, 72
BPAs & Plastics, 165
Bringing up children, *23*
Brucie Bonus, 90
Bullet Proof Coffees, *89*

Burn More Calories, *82*
Burnt Foods, 166
business, 49
butane, 63

C

Cancer, *15*
Carpets & Curtains (VOCs), 166
cartilage, *125*
Check the Label, *143*
chemicals, *68*
chronic disease, *16*
chronic illness, *16*
Cold Shower, *145*
Collagen, *125*
Commuting, *24*
cortisol, *25*
cryotherapy, *6*
Cryotherapy Chamber, *6*, *164*
Cryotherapy Chambers, 165
cutting-edge treatments, *10*

D

Daily Routine., 36
Daily Routines, 43
deep sleep, 95
Diabetes, *15*, *76*
diet, 73
Diethanolamine (DEA), *64*
Directors and Partners of companies, 1
Disinfectant sprays, *58*
DMDM Hydantoin, *64*
DON'T EAT IT, 109
doubts, 115

Drinking Alcohol, 155

E

Eat Early, 153
electrical devices, 102
Electro & Magnetic Field Radiation, 151
ELF (extremely low frequency), *65*
emergencies, *21*
EMF (electromagnetic fields), *59*
EMF radiation, 59
Environment, 36
Exercise, *9*
Extremely Hot Environments, 145

F

Farming, *68*
Fasting, *9*
Fat Freezing Machine, *6*
Fibromyalgia, *76*
fluoride, *62*
Fluoride, 166
Foam Bedding, 166
Food Additives., 166
forest bathing, *32*

G

genome, 124
Get Outside, 150
Give me 10 (years), 149
Give Me 5 (years), 143
glucose, *25*
Gratitude, 148

H

Health worries, *23*
heart disease, *16*
Heart disease, *15*
heightened risk, *25*

HIFEM Accelerated Muscle Stimulation device, *6*
HIFU Machine, *6*
hormones, *25*
Hydrogen peroxide, *58*
hyperbaric oxygen chamber, *6*
Hyperbaric Oxygen Chamber, *6*
hyperbaric oxygen therapy, *6*
Hyperbaric Oxygen Therapy Chambers, 165
Hyperthyroidism, *76*

I

immune system, *16*
Improve - Exercise, *111*
Improve - Infrastructure, *117*
Improve - Mind, *131*
Improve - Nutrients, *109*
Improve - Sleep, *95*
Improved Alertness, *82*
Improves Your Circulation, 81
Increased Willpower, *82*
inflammation, *15*
Intermittent Hypoxia Therapy., 165

J

job, 24
Joint Pain, *124*
joints, *117*, 124

L

labels of food, *21*
Lead Piping, 166
leukocytes production, *82*
ligaments, *117*
Localised Cryotherapy Device, *6*
longevity coaching, *6*
Longevity Coaching, *161*
Lung disease, *15*

M

McDonald's iced frappe, *21*
Menopause, *77*
mental wellbeing, *24*
Mercury, *72*
Metal work, *68*
Mineral oil, *64*
Mining, *68*
modern western world, *26*
Monoethanolamine (MEA), *64*
MSGs (Mono sodium glutamate), 166
MSGs (monosodium glutamate), *74*
Multiple Sclerosis, *76*
muscles, *117*

N

Nail technicians, *68*
Neighbours, 55
nutrients, *109*
Nutrients, 155
nutshell, 81

O

offgassing, *67*
Optimistic, 136
outraged, *23*
Overview, 11
Oxygen Facial Device, *6*

P

PAHs (Polycyclic Aromatic Hydrocarbons), *73*
painkillers, *84*
Paint, 166
Parabens, *64*
Patek Phillipe watches, *12*
PE (physical education), *62*
Pesticides., 165
physical wellbeing, *24*

phytoncide, *32*
Plastic Manufacturing, *68*
PMA, *131*
PMS, *76*
pollution, *76*
Polyethyline glycol, *64*
Problematic People, *144*
Propylene Glycol (PG), *64*

R

Red Light Therapy, *6*
Red Light Therapy., 165
reduction, *19*
Remove - Calories, *83*
Remove - Heat, *75*
Remove - Stress, *23*
Remove - Sugar, *15*
Remove - Toxins, *35*
Removing and Improving, *9*
rheumatoid arthritis, *25*
Rolls Royce convertibles, *12*
Rubber manufacturing, *68*

S

shagging at 90!, *36*
sick building syndrome, *65*
silent killer, *24*
silent killers, *15*
skeletal structure, *117*
Skin Care Toxins, 166
Sleep, *9*
Sleep Mastery, *161*
Sleep Quality, *102*
soft drink, *19*
Soft/Soda Drinks, *143*
Stiff Muscles, *126*
Stop Killing Yourself, *9*
Stress, *9*
Stress & Anxiety, *76*
Stressful jobs in general, *68*
Strokes, *15*

sugar, *19*
Sugar, *9*
Sweet Snacks, *143*
Sweeteners, 165
symptoms, *24*
Synthetic fragrances, *64*

T

Tap Water Contaminants, 166
The Best Beds in the World, 165
The Longevity Clinic, *6*, *159*
The Profitable Clinic, *7*
The Skin Repair Group, *7*, *75*
The Skin Repair Pen, *6*
thyroid hormone production, *72*
tobacco companies, *65*
Top 5 Super Removers, *54*
toxic anti-social media, *26*
toxins, *68*
Toxins, *9*
Trans Fats, *73*
Triclosan, *64*
Triethanolamine (TEA), *64*

U

Uptight and sensitive people, 2

US Environmental Protection Agency
  (EPA), *67*
UV lights., 166

V

Vegetable & Seed Oils, 73
veins, 81
Victorians, *56*

W

Washing detergent, 166
Water, 69
What's New Pussy Cat!, 93
WIFI & Mobile Phones., 166
Work deadlines, *23*

Y

yacht, *12*
You Are What You Think You Are..., 135
You Glow, 82
youngevity, *10*
Your Personalised Longevity Plan, 139
Your Toxic Checklist, 37
Youth Mastery, *161*

TROUBLE SLEEPING?
MY NEXT WORKBOOK WAS
WRITTEN FOR YOU…

STOP!!
WAKING UP
TIRED...

THE BEGINNERS GUIDE TO SLEEP

AVAILABLE NOW

FEELING STRESSED?
MY NEXT WORKBOOK WAS
WRITTEN FOR YOU…

STOP!!
STRESSING OUT...

THE BEGINNERS GUIDE TO STRESS

COMING IN SPRING 2024